The Vitamin Solution

TWO DOCTORS CLEAR THE CONFUSION ABOUT VITAMINS AND YOUR HEALTH

The Vitamin Solution

TWO DOCTORS CLEAR THE CONFUSION ABOUT VITAMINS AND YOUR HEALTH

ARIELLE LEVITAN, MD,
& ROMY BLOCK, MD

SHE WRITES PRESS

Published 2015
Printed in the United States of America
ISBN: 978-1-63152-014-3

Library of Congress Control Number: 2015947338

For information, address:
She Writes Press
1563 Solano Ave #546
Berkeley, CA 94707

She Writes Press is a division of SparkPoint Studio, LLC.

DEDICATION

To our mothers, Renee and Susan,
for always having only the
highest expectations for us
and instilling in us the drive
to create something better.

TABLE OF CONTENTS

Part Three: Vitamins for Prevention

Part Four: Beyond Vitamins

Part Five: Final Thoughts

INTRODUCTION
NOT SURE THIS BOOK
IS FOR YOU? READ THIS . . .

IF YOU KNOW WITH 100 PERCENT CERTAINTY what exact amounts of which exact type and source of vitamins you do and don't need to take every day for the rest of your life in order to live the healthiest, longest, most incredibly awesome and uplifting life, you can stop reading this right now.

However, if you are like the rest of us and have felt somewhat confused about vitamins, we suggest you read on.

If you want to learn the medically sound, experientially proven truth about what vitamins are necessary, useful, and important for your health, then you are in the right place.

If you want to find out what commonly sold vitamins are potentially harmful to your health and well-being, then please read on.

By following us through our journey of the last fifteen or so years, you will get the wisdom we have attained—through medical school, residency, and fellowship training; taking care of thousands of patients; culling through the medical and lay literature; and talking to friends, family, nutritionists, trainers, and just about everyone you can imagine—served up to you in a simple, concise format.

You will no longer be confused about vitamins. You will in fact have a much clearer picture about how vitamins relate to your unique health needs. You will have a game plan to start on your journey to finding your best health. Join us as we begin.

Who We Are

We are you. We are two women, with husbands, with children, who happen to have MDs after our names. We are also two women who were at one time confused and overwhelmed by all of the information coming at us about vitamins.

Romy Block is a practicing endocrinologist. She hails from Highland Park, Illinois, where she lives with her husband, Adam (also a doctor—a pulmonary, critical care, and sleep specialist), and their three very active boys. Romy journeyed far from her Chicago home, only to eventually find her way back. She and Adam met in Israel while in medical school at Tel Aviv University. She completed her undergraduate studies at Tufts University and her residency at North Shore University Hospital, North Shore-LIJ. Her fellowship in endocrinology and metabolism was at New York University. Phew . . . that's a lot of years of training.

Arielle Miller Levitan grew up in Princeton, New Jersey, but now resides around the corner from Romy, with her husband, Victor (a doctor of internal medicine, just like she is), and their three challenging but wonderful adolescents. Arielle did her undergraduate work at Stanford University and then made the Midwest her home at Northwestern University's Feinberg School of Medicine. She did her training in internal medicine at Northwestern's Evanston Hospital program.

We met through work, but became fast friends when we realized we had so many things in common. We lived around the corner from each other, and both of us had doctor husbands and three kids. As our friendship grew, we would often take long walks for exercise and rehash stories about our families and our experiences as doctors.

One subject that came up again and again was vitamins. It seemed that every patient either of us saw had some confusion about what they should be taking. As a primary care doctor, Arielle spends much of her time advising patients about what they should be taking to feel better, protect and strengthen their bones, and prevent illness. As a specialist in endocrinology and metabolism, Romy sees people every day with complaints about weight gain, fatigue, and thinning hair, who often think they have a thyroid or adrenal issue. Upon further investigation, Romy often finds that these people do not have a glandular problem; rather they have nutritional deficiencies that are causing their symptoms.

As physicians, we had the tools to educate ourselves about vitamins. We were able to go from clueless medical students to experienced doctors over a several-decade journey. During this time we were able to research the medical data and talk to other experts in a variety of specialties. And, perhaps most importantly, we have had the benefit of treating thousands of patients and hearing their stories and experiences.

We have learned over the years that vitamins are an essential part of health for all of us. Some can be obtained from what we eat, others cannot. The challenge is figuring out which person needs what vitamins. And, in fact, the answer is rarely the same for two people. We are all different. We do not eat the same, exercise the same, or live the same. We all have unique health histories and life circumstances.

In 2014 we cofounded a company called Vous Vitamin, LLC based on this very premise. We wanted to create a means by which people anywhere could do a simple online survey and get a multivitamin tailored to their needs. We could not find safe, high-quality products to recommend to our patients so we created them. Our system has given people everywhere the ability to get exactly what vitamins they need at their particular stage in life.

Through this process we have learned an immense amount about vitamins and health. Join us as we take you through what we have learned over the years so you can find out exactly what you need to embark on a journey toward finding your best health.

The Confusion

It started in our youth with the good old Flintstones™ Chewables. Why were we supposed to take them? Did everyone have to? Some kids did, others didn't. Romy remembers her mother asking the doctor, and he said, "It can't hurt." Is that really true? We never knew. They tasted kind of good at first, like candy, but then not so good as they went down. At what age does one stop taking them? Hmm . . .

The confusion continued into our college years, when no one was doing much about anything to take care of themselves, but a few lone friends swore that vitamins were the key to pulling all-nighters and hangover recovery. If other friends took them, we never knew about it. And then medical school began. Arielle remembers in detail the single two-hour lecture in med school on nutrition. The registered dietician who gave the lecture said, "This may be the only chance you get to learn this stuff, but you will literally need it every day of your life." She could not have been more correct. The saddest part is that really was the only time in medical school or residency that nutrition was given the spotlight. The lecture was useful, but seemed far less glamorous than topics like treating heart attacks, broken bones, or overwhelming infections. We both put the topic of vitamins and nutrition on the back burner for a few years, while we learned the ins and outs of treating "real" disease.

Perhaps neither of us realized so early on in our medical training that treating disease really starts long before the person shows up in the emergency room gravely ill. Treating that broken hip in a seventy-five-year-old woman actually starts in her thirties by giving her the correct nutrients to prevent that fracture so many years later. We were young and foolish, wrapped up in the excitement and the very necessary focus on treating the seriously ill.

As time went on, we each settled into our specialties and our practices. We refined our skills in treating common ailments and we spent over a decade each seeing patients, always working to find out how best to treat their symptoms and to prevent future problems.

Over the years, we came to realize that just about every patient we see has issues related to vitamins. They want to know if they need to take vitamins and, if so, which ones. Often they fear they may require major medication or interventions, which can frequently be addressed by correcting nutritional deficiencies. Almost always, we want to partner with them to help prevent future health problems, which often involves a combination of lifestyle modification and dietary supplementation. We see patients who pull big bags full of bottles out of their purses, saying, "My neighbor said to take this and my hair stylist said to take this." We also, sadly, see patients in the intensive care unit (ICU) with grave health conditions caused by taking the wrong products. This is a widespread problem and serious business.

The overarching theme is confusion. No one knows what to take that is both safe and useful. As doctors, we were uncertain of these answers when we first embarked on our careers. We have each spent many years, individually and ultimately together, researching vitamins, the data, and the myths. We've also spent years talking to our patients in great detail about what they have taken, why they took it, and how it affected them. We have toured vitamin manufacturers' plants and headquarters, learned about their processes, and seen firsthand what practices can and should be employed to guarantee high-quality, pure products. New research is constantly coming out, and we work hard to stay on top of it. We have also spent many years culling through what is out there, to determine what products in what form are truly beneficial and safe.

Perhaps most importantly, we have learned that we are not all the same. All of our needs are not the same. We each possess a unique combination of factors (diet, health history, genetics, symptoms, and lifestyle choices) that makes our needs individual. We have found ways to tailor our nutritional advice to individuals based on their particular needs. The person who feels great does not always need the same vitamins as the person who is fatigued or who has hair that is thinning.

The culmination of our many years of learning lies in these pages.

PART ONE: SETTING THE STAGE

CHAPTER 1
IMPROVING YOUR HEALTH

Failure is not fatal, but failure to change might be.
—JOHN WOODEN

It does not matter how slowly you go so long as you do not stop.
—CONFUCIUS

THERE IS ALWAYS AN EXCUSE. Work. Kids. Household responsibilities. Tending to a spouse. Caring for aging parents. You can easily fill all the hours of the day with things other than taking care of yourself. Whether your goal is to lose weight, stop smoking, eat more healthfully, exercise more regularly, or all of the above, these changes *can* be made if you want to make them. We would like to help you get in the proper frame of mind.

What to Change?

This will be further outlined later in the book. We will give you specific strategies, largely through the use of basic lifestyle modifications, dietary changes, and some simple vitamin solutions. As you read further, you will choose which aspects of your life you would like to improve—from sleep to exercise to diet to health habits.

Why Change?

Perhaps the same reasons that hold you back from changing are the very reason you should in fact take these steps. In other words, you care so much about the other people in your life; it is for this reason that you should care for your own health. You spend so much time and effort raising your own children, but you will not be able to continue doing so if your own health is compromised. Think long term here (even grandchildren). Your career can also be enhanced by better health. Your improved physical stamina will help you perform maximally at work mentally, and your improved overall health will enhance your ability to focus and succeed. Your healthier look will draw people to you even if it is on a subconscious level.

We challenge you to take the time and effort to make your own health a priority. If you are reading this book you have already shown that you have interest in obtaining the necessary knowledge. But we all know people who watch the Food Network incessantly but never actually cook. Don't be that person. Be the person who actually puts the knowledge to use.

Make a Deal with Yourself

We don't mean something like, "If I lose fifty pounds, I will go on a trip to Hawaii." Rather, make a deal to embrace the idea of progress and improvement. Commit to commitment. This includes the failures that will inevitably come with it. You will not always reach a specific goal when you want to reach it. However, if you have an overall level of dedication to the process, you will use each failure to learn something about yourself and ultimately to push yourself forward.

The commitment is not as big as you think—no matter how bad your diet or lifestyle habits are. *The only vow necessary to take is to do better than you are doing right now.*

The Psychology of Change: The Dental-Floss Principle

Drastic change does not always work. What does work is slow incremental change that moves you gradually closer to your ideal goal. Molding your daily habits over a period of months to years will ultimately add up to seismic change if you continually make adjustments in the right direction.

We have all been guilty of not flossing enough. We've been chided by the dentist year after year about the importance of flossing every day. However, it is the one time that the dentist asks you, "Why don't you try flossing every other day?" that you think, "I can do that." It alleviates the pressure.

The same holds true for exercise. If you are not a regular exerciser, the thought of embarking on a routine can be overwhelming to say the least. You see all those "health nuts" around you doing triathlons or spending hours at the gym. Not happening, right?

That is not what you need to use as your goal. Use the dental-floss principle. Something is better than nothing. Your initial exercise routine can consist of ten minutes a day of simple, at-home exercises or walking. *The New York Times'* "Scientific 7-Minute Workout" is an intense program that literally takes seven minutes a day. We warn you, it is not easy and may require some ramping up to, but who can't spare seven minutes?

Goal Setting

Just as flossing every other day, rather than every day, is much less daunting, giving yourself simple, attainable goals can give you permission to make some of the positive changes that you know you need.

Eliminate one bad food from your diet, or one time of day when you tend to overindulge, commit to staying in control. You will not drop fifty pounds in a month this way (nor should you; it will never stay off), but you will make small progress. Perhaps more importantly, you will get a taste of success. You will show yourself that changing habits is possible and you will give yourself permission to continue to make changes, small as they may be.

Plan to Have a Plan

The good news about adopting a plan is you already have the framework in place. Don't think so? You really do. You already have some structure to your daily life that serves as the basis for molding your behaviors.

Even something as routine and simple as brushing your teeth can be paired with another activity. In fact, the more routine the behavior, the better. If you tell yourself in advance that you will not brush your teeth until you do ten pushups, this is an easy mechanism to ensure that you do ten pushups a day (or ultimately twice a day, depending upon your goal). The change will be best remembered if you tie a ribbon on your toothbrush or make some other form of a reminder paired with the habit. We often tell our customers who purchase daily Personalized Multivitamins™ to keep their vitamins on top of their coffeemaker if this is part of their daily ritual.

So set some incremental goals. One plan may be to not let yourself shower for the day until you have exercised. Not a morning person? Make exercising on a treadmill or stationary bike part of your evening TV-watching routine. Don't have the money or the space for at-home cardio equipment? Get a workout DVD, walk or run outside, or see our fitness tips in the Exercise chapter for lots of inexpensive, easy ways to exercise at home. Whatever means of exercise you choose, tie your intended activity with a regular (hopefully enjoyable) habit. You can then manipulate the length of your activity gradually over time. Fifteen minutes of exercise can extend to twenty, increasing by a minute each day.

Make getting your mammogram or going to the doctor part of a girls' day shopping or going to the spa. What better way to celebrate your friendship than to make sure that you are each taking care of your own health? Likewise, turn your lunch date into a walking date. Keep each other accountable.

Dietary changes can also be tied to existing routines. You can plan to continue eating multiple enjoyable meals each day, but with advanced planning, you can replace some less healthful habits with better ones. Your usual fast-food lunch can be replaced with a healthful lunch packed at home or a purchased salad, with an enjoyable treat built in for after lunch (three Hershey's Kisses or some other satisfying but well-portioned treat). Or the reward can be slightly delayed to help get you through the day. A healthful lunch can be rewarded with a small frozen yogurt treat in the afternoon (perhaps replacing that bag of candy you typically have at that time).

Replacing bad habits with good can also have a powerful effect. For example, quitting smoking can be paired with starting an exercise routine. This helps for many reasons: It may replace your time when you might be smoking with something else to keep you busy. Instead of the after-dinner cigarette, make it an after-dinner walk around the block. The exercise also helps combat the weight gain that can sometimes accompany quitting tobacco. Likewise, instead of going to the store to purchase cigarettes, put the money you would have spent in a jar each day. When you reach a target amount, go buy yourself a coveted item.

Does this sound like a child's sticker chart for good behavior posted on the fridge? It might. But that is okay, because it works. It gives you positive feedback on your good behaviors. Even the most disciplined of us need that to keep us moving forward.

As you work toward achieving various health goals, vitamins can play a crucial role in any comprehensive health regimen. They too require some planning and discipline. And, of course, knowing what to take to best suit your needs is the key! More on that later . . .

Maintenance Plan

Reaching a goal can be thrilling and invigorating. But stopping our actions at that point can defeat the entire purpose. This is perhaps most typically seen in those who have a goal weight they want to achieve. They get to the goal and then stop all the great habits that got them there in the first place. This will not be you if you have a maintenance plan in place, before you reach your goal. Your changes are part of a lifestyle that you will continue to maintain moving forward. You must build that new lifestyle into a long-term plan. Establish means to check in on your habits, either with continued weigh-ins or set plans. For example, after you run the half-marathon, make sure you are signed up for another race, or have some alternative form of exercise already scheduled so you keep up the momentum. The key here is having these plans made *before* you reach your goal, so the future becomes part of the process.

As you look toward bettering your health, questions about vitamins often arise. When you are considering diet, nutrition, and exercise, vitamins can and often should play into the equation. Next we will start to delve into their important role.

CHAPTER 2
VITAMIN MYTHS

PATIENTS OFTEN COME IN AND ASK whether they should be taking vitamins. Many are already taking something; many are not. The answer is never simple, because this is NOT a yes-or-no question. It comes down to analyzing their exact circumstances to determine what they should be taking.

One of the reasons that this question comes up so often is that there has been a great deal in the press recently regarding multivitamins and their effects or possible lack thereof. And there is good reason for this concern. The large studies that have been done have failed to demonstrate that people they assigned to take multivitamins actually lived longer.

But these studies are flawed for many reasons. Firstly, the groups that were allegedly taking the vitamins often were not really taking them. This is one of the greatest difficulties in studying vitamin use. People often stop taking them. Sometimes it is for valid reasons such as side effects, or cost. Sometimes they just stop. They often do so because they lose faith that the pill is "doing anything," largely because the effects of vitamins take many months to see or feel, and some effects you may never actually feel (such as stronger bones or not getting a condition you might have otherwise developed). Therefore, to accurately say that this group of "vitamin takers" did not have longer lives is rather inaccurate. We don't know what would have happened if they did not take the pills—their health could have been even worse. A more recent 2015 study in the *Journal of Nutrition* did show a mortality benefit. Women who took a multivitamin for more than three years did have a lower death rate from cardiac causes. So we may have more to learn about exactly who benefits from vitamins and under what circumstances.

Interestingly, the outcomes these studies measured can also be questioned. Just looking at "all-cause mortality," i.e., death rates, is not terribly helpful. There is something to be said for quality of life, disease prevention, treatment of symptoms, and other possible effects of vitamin use.

Perhaps the most major flaw is to assume that thousands and thousands of people would all be served by taking any generic off-the-shelf combination of vitamins. How could every one of these people have the same needs?

For that reason, we will begin by delving into different issues and the role of vitamins in health. We will then discuss individual vitamins, who may benefit from taking them, and why. As for our original question, "Should I be taking vitamins?" The answer is likely "yes" and "no." Yes you should, but perhaps not the typical concoctions you find at your corner pharmacy. You likely need more of certain things and less of others, and this largely depends on who exactly you are. So read on to find out what you do and don't need.

Some Common Misperceptions: Six Myths about Vitamins

VITAMIN MYTH #1: TAKING A MULTIVITAMIN IS OF NO USE.

As mentioned previously, a recent study compared a large group of people taking a generic, off-the-shelf multivitamin to a group who was not taking a vitamin. The study found that the group taking the vitamins did not live longer than the other group. From that, the "vitamins are of no benefit to you" myth was affirmed. We do not believe the study disproves the value of vitamins for all individuals. We believe the study is not helpful for many reasons—one being that generic, off-the-shelf multivitamins contain too little of many of the nutrients most of us need, while they may contain too much of certain ingredients, which may be harmful at those levels. The takeaway should be that not all people or their vitamins are created equal. Many people *can* benefit from the appropriate combination of vitamins. Figuring out what vitamins *you* should take, based on your individual diet, health history, and lifestyle, is the important part.

VITAMIN MYTH #2: I CAN TAKE LOTS OF VITAMINS AND MY BODY WILL JUST ABSORB WHAT IT NEEDS, THE REST WILL JUST NOT BE ABSORBED.

Actually, certain vitamins can harm you in high doses. Specifically, fat-soluble vitamins (i.e., those that hang around for a long time in your system because they are incorporated into the fatty parts of your cells—typically in the liver) such as vitamin D, vitamin E, vitamin A, and vitamin K can cause toxicity if you take excessive doses. Symptoms of vitamin overdoses include severe headaches, bad skin, liver function abnormalities, and many other consequences. One large study also suggested that even moderate doses of vitamin A can increase rates of cancer in certain populations. Likewise excessive heavy metals may play a role in certain liver diseases and dementias such as Alzheimer's. Almost any vitamin in high enough doses can cause problems. Don't overdo it—getting enough, but not too much, is the goal.

VITAMIN MYTH #3: ALL BRANDS OF VITAMINS ARE EQUIVALENT. IF THEY ARE SOLD IN THE STORE, THEY MUST BE SAFE.

Unfortunately, the vitamin manufacturing process is not regulated by the Food and Drug Administration (FDA) in the same way that prescription and other over-the-counter medications are. Therefore, quality control in the supplement industry can be poor. Studies analyzing off-the-shelf vitamins and supplements have shown that some products contain contaminants and other unlisted ingredients that can cause serious health problems. In fact, a recent analysis of commonly sold herbal supplements found little to none of the claimed ingredients in the actual products. This leads one to wonder, what then is in them and what harm can they cause?

Part of our goal in cofounding Vous Vitamin® was to give people access to a reputable, high-quality brand that adheres to extremely high manufacturing standards. Our manufacturer holds National Sanitation Foundation (NSF) certification and is licensed and regularly inspected for good manufacturing practices (GMP) by state and federal health authorities to ensure compliance. Looking for these, as well U.S. Pharmacopeial Convention (USP) certification, are good ways to monitor products for their quality and purity.

VITAMIN MYTH #4: MY DOCTOR WILL TELL ME WHAT VITAMINS I SHOULD TAKE.

Doctors will often take the time to discuss your specific vitamin needs. However, we know from experience, there is not always an opportunity to go through a detailed analysis of your diet and lifestyle at a routine visit. Also, many doctors hesitate to make recommendations about vitamins because they are concerned about recommending products that are not FDA regulated and they cannot be certain you will take a well-made, quality brand. Sometimes physicians will check certain vitamin levels as part of your visit. But, these can be costly and often not necessary, since a detailed history will usually reveal what deficiencies you may have. Unfortunately, our current medical system does not make this discussion an important part of our healthcare delivery. Our current model of health care tends to emphasize treating existing conditions with prescription medications rather than preventing them in the first place or using more natural remedies to treat problems.

VITAMIN MYTH #5: IF I EAT A HEALTHFUL DIET, I PROBABLY DO NOT NEED ANY VITAMINS.

While it is *possible* to get everything you need via diet, it is not probable that you do. For example, people who eat a lot of fruits and vegetables get many essential nutrients (e.g., vitamin A, vitamin C, etc.), but tend to eat less of certain other nutrients (like vitamin B12 and iron found in red meat). Additionally, certain vitamins are hard to come by in most diets. Vitamin D3 is one such vitamin. It is only found in a few food sources at a significant levels, such as wild-caught salmon (not farm raised). Consider the iodine dilemma of the healthy eater. In avoiding processed foods and using natural sea salt or kosher salt, the healthy eater may be missing out on the recommended daily allowance of iodine (found in iodized salt)—which is essential for thyroid health and metabolism.

VITAMIN MYTH #6: I SHOULD ALWAYS TAKE THE SAME VITAMINS.

If your diet and lifestyle varies significantly from month to month or day to day, your needs will naturally change. You should reevaluate your daily vitamin routine at least every six to twelve months as your health and nutrient intake evolves. Likewise, certain days may call for extra boosts in certain vitamins. Taking an as-needed dose of certain nutrients at specific times may be useful. For example, an intense workout or excessive alcohol intake may require more electrolytes and B vitamins to combat the losses. Feeling run down or coming down with a cold may call for some zinc and extra vitamin C and D for immune support.

CHAPTER 3
VITAMIN HORROR STORIES

OVER THE YEARS OF SEEING THOUSANDS of patients, we have heard so much wonderful feedback, often about benefits they have seen from taking different vitamins and supplements. We have unfortunately also seen many negative effects and some downright tragedies.

These horror stories often occur when people listen to untrustworthy sources (and the Internet is chock-full of them—how can one know whom to trust on what to take? Also, they may recommend taking vitamins in improper doses). There can also be untoward and lethal effects from taking products that are contaminated with other additives. These are not always listed on the label. Unfortunately, vitamin manufacturing is not FDA regulated and many manufacturers' quality-control processes are far from perfect. Ingredients may be sourced from China or other non-U.S. sources, and their contents not verified or assessed for quality and purity. This is an industry where a trustworthy source is essential!

The following five cases illustrate what we mean.

Case #1: Too much of a good thing is not better

A forty-two-year-old woman feels down during the long winter months. She consults with an online holistic doctor who says her symptoms are likely due to vitamin D deficiency. He advises she start a high-dose supplement to treat her symptoms. Under his advisement, she begins taking 10,000 international units (IUs) of vitamin D3 daily. Within a few weeks she feels somewhat better, less sad and more energetic. This however, is short-lived. She becomes increasingly fatigued, lethargic, and constipated. About six weeks after starting this new regimen, her husband has to call 911 because she is barely arousable. She has in fact overdosed on vitamin D, which causes her parathyroid/calcium regulatory system to go off-kilter. Heavy doses of vitamin D cause massive amounts of serum calcium to accumulate, which in turn results in a near-comatose state and other complications. After a weeklong ICU stay, the effects are ultimately reversed.

Vitamin D in massive doses can be toxic. It is a fat-soluble vitamin that over time accumulates in your body. However, in reasonable daily doses the majority of us benefit from it and in fact need it in supplement form. Knowing (based on where you live, your diet, and other factors) what a reasonable daily dosage is the important thing here. Also, realizing that treating vitamin D deficiency is a slow process that does not happen over weeks, but rather months, is essential. Lesson learned, we hope.

Case #2: Not so smooth move

A twenty-five-year-old law student struggles with constipation. She only moves her bowels every two to three days and feels bloated, gassy, and uncomfortable in between. A friend advises her to take some "natural" supplements from a local health food store. They include: milkweed and Siberian ginseng. Twenty-four hours later her constipation symptoms persist, and she becomes dizzy and lightheaded. Evaluation in the emergency room reveals a dangerously high potassium level from the products she ingested. The high potassium causes cardiac issues and arrhythmias until she is treated with the proper intravenous (IV) medications.

What was actually in these health store products and at what exact dose is still uncertain. After ruling out all other variables, it is clear the "natural" supplements caused some potentially life-threatening side effects. The patient is fortunate to be treated quickly.

Case #3: Anxious to feel better

A fifty-three-year-old woman has a long history of anxiety and depression treated with commonly prescribed medication. She feels her medication is no longer working as well as it should be, so she consults with a naturopath who says she has a low level of T3 (a form of thyroid hormone) despite the fact that her regular doctor said her thyroid tests are normal. She starts taking a "natural" thyroid replacement (a "glandular" preparation of T3, made from animal thyroid). For the next few weeks she finds she feels energetic in the morning after taking her T3 but completely exhausted in the afternoons. The naturopath says she has "adrenal fatigue" and adds a didehydroepiandrosterone (DHEA) supplement and St. John's wort. Three weeks later she ends up hospitalized for palpitations, tremors, muscle cramping, and diarrhea. She is found to have "serotonin syndrome," triggered by starting the addition of these new "natural" products. The T3 has also caused her to be hyperthyroid and contributes to her symptoms as well.

The combination of certain supplements with some prescribed medications can cause significant harm. Additionally, the use of "natural glandular replacements" can be both unnecessary and dangerous. These products are often made from ground-up pig or cow glands. The concentrations found in different batches are erratic and often toxic.

Case #4: Not so energetic

A thirty-one-year-old man drinks several energy drinks early one morning to combat feeling tired after a late night of drinking. He then spends much of the day doing physical activity both at the gym and then outdoors playing sports with friends. While playing in a pickup basketball game, he collapses and the paramedics are called. He is found to have extreme dehydration and muscle breakdown (a condition known as rhabdomyolysis). This then causes kidney damage when broken-down muscle floods the kidneys. Aggressive hydration and treatment in the ICU ultimately reverses the damage. Most likely, the large doses of caffeine found in the energy drinks contributed to his extreme dehydration and gave him a false sense of energy throughout the day.

Case #5: Doctor does not always know best

A thirty-six-year-old woman is told by her family doctor that she has high cholesterol. She mentions this to her chiropractor, who then advises she try taking niacin, a B vitamin for lowering cholesterol. She begins taking the dosage he advised and provided to her. Within two weeks she feels poorly and notes abdominal pain, nausea, vomiting, dark urine, and her skin color is yellow. She develops severe hepatitis and liver failure due to the supplement. She is transferred from her community hospital to a major medical center for liver transplantation.

Enough said.

These cases are not intended to scare you to death and make you never want to take a vitamin or supplement again. Rather, they are meant to illustrate that these products, if used improperly, can have serious ramifications. Just because something is sold over the counter doesn't mean it can't have potentially major side effects.

Here are a few takeaway messages when it comes to vitamins and supplements:

- Make sure you are taking pure, well-made products from a reputable source. GMP, USP and NSF certification can be a useful way to ensure higher quality.
- Make sure products are taken in appropriate doses.
- Make sure products do not have potential interactions with other medications or supplements.
- Review concerns with your physician and do not fail to mention over-the-counter products that you are taking at your doctor's visits.

Bettering your health is clearly not a one-step process. We have talked about ways to further motivate yourself toward change. We have also discussed some techniques to make sure that you meet your goals by having a mindset that includes a total lifestyle approach, rather than just a goal weight or short-term plan.

Looking globally at your habits and health should involve a consideration of vitamins and their role. This is no simple answer; there are many factors that each individual needs to consider when weighing his or her vitamin options. Safety and avoiding danger are of the utmost concern, as you probably can see from the horror stories above (as the Hippocratic Oath goes, "First, do no harm"). Then it is essential to look at yourself as a whole person (made up of your diet, lifestyle, and health issues) to start figuring out what vitamins are both necessary and useful to you going forward.

PART TWO:
VITAMINS FOR
SPECIFIC AILMENTS

CHAPTER 4
ENERGY AND FATIGUE

IF WE HAD TO COME UP with the most common complaint from our patients, fatigue and lack of energy would be it. It seems that just about everyone we see feels, at least some of the time, more tired than they should be.

Feeling energetic and well-rested can make or break just about every aspect of our lives, including our health, productivity at work, even our home life and relationships. Sometimes when people get into a downward spiral, their lack of energy makes it hard to take care of themselves properly, and that only worsens the problem. Unraveling all of these issues is essential to remedying them.

The background for energy- and fatigue-related complaints varies a great deal by stage of life:

- **The young singles** (twenty-somethings) tend to "burn the candle at both ends" by overdoing it at work and play. They stay out too late, drink too much, eat less than healthfully, work long hours, and then expect to start all over again the next day. They may "recover" on the weekend by sleeping in and exercising, but healthy living is the exception more than the rule.

- **The parental set** are the parents of younger children who feel like they are running on an endless treadmill, exhausted all the time. They are up frequently at night with their children and have little time to themselves after work and child care responsibilities are done. They feed their exhaustion with kid-friendly, unhealthful snacks, and they tend to neglect their own health at the expense of doing everything for everyone else.

- **The forty- and fifty-somethings** have replaced changing diapers with a new set of stressors. Career responsibilities peak as parenting older tween, teen, and young adult children bring on new challenges. They may also be assuming care for aging parents. Middle-aged people notice they have more trouble sleeping and take longer to recover from minor illnesses and injuries. They also feel the effects of alcohol and caffeine more significantly.

- **The Medicare set** find they struggle with sleep. They awaken too early and find that daily activities take more out of them than they once did. They have more time to devote to taking care of themselves, but more ailments to boot.

The above generalizations about each cohort are just that. Of course, individuals at any given stage of life may have vastly different experiences. These profiles are simply common ones that we see. Why is this important?

Each of these stages is marked by *habits and patterns* that contribute to feeling fatigued and lackluster. They are modifiable behaviors and remediable symptoms that can be improved by a combination of lifestyle changes and replenishment of missing nutrients.

Start with the Obvious: Sleep

No discussion about fatigue—or health for that matter—would be complete without a mention of sleep. Sleep is so essential to human vitality that research now shows it is linked to just about every aspect of our health. Find out more about sleep and its essential role in energy and fatigue in our Sleep chapter.

Our purposes in this chapter, however, are to highlight the key role that vitamins can play in humans' energy levels. Many common vitamins are essential in making our various cells function properly;

by contrast, deficiencies in our levels of all the following vitamins can cause a lack of energy:

IRON

One of the most classic causes of low energy is iron deficiency. This is a very common issue today, particularly in women. Women's bodies are constantly shifting and changing. Iron loss is a normal part of this cycle. We require more iron during pregnancy and while nursing our children. Those who get menstrual periods regularly lose blood and iron with menstruation. Heavier periods account for even more iron loss. All of these factors add up. Childbearing and monthly menses can deplete women's iron stores for years to follow.

Men too can be iron deficient due to insufficient amounts of iron in their diets. Some men and women can have unknown (or "occult") blood losses through their gastrointestinal (GI) tracts, such as bleeding ulcers or colon polyps. These issues need to be addressed by a physician.

Another group of people who tend to lack iron are those with GI problems that limit absorption. This includes people with celiac disease, inflammatory bowel disease (IBD, such as Crohn's or colitis), or people who have had gastric surgeries such as gastric bypass for obesity.

Why is iron so important? It is used by your body to hold on to oxygen in your blood and transport it to your tissues. At the cellular level, iron is used to make energy and to fuel enzymes.

You may wonder, "Wouldn't my doctor know if I was iron deficient?" The answer is, not always. Routine blood testing usually includes a complete blood count (CBC). This includes the hemoglobin and hematocrit levels, i.e., the amount of cells that are made from iron and are used by the blood to transport oxygen and other nutrients all over the body. Low hemoglobin or hematocrit levels are known as anemia, which is often the result of severe iron deficiency. Earlier stages of iron deficiency require special testing of specific iron levels and ferritin levels, which reflect how much iron your body has stored up.

Many people with iron deficiency (even at the early stages, not yet detectable in a blood count) report symptoms of fatigue, brain fog, lack of energy, depression, and even hair loss. Therefore, replacing this important element is essential.

Then how do we replace the iron? Some of us replenish our iron from a well-rounded diet. However, the American diet has changed significantly over the last few decades. Our "healthier diet," geared toward prevention of heart disease, now contains significantly less red meat than it once did. Most of us are eating red meat much less frequently than we used to. Fabulous as this may be for our cholesterol and heart health, it has actually contributed to widespread iron deficiency.

While some vegetables are iron sources, they have lower amounts and are not as well absorbed. Therefore, vegetarians are at high risk for iron deficiency. Other contributing risks are antacids and stomach medications for inflammation, which can also decrease your iron absorption. That means you may not actually be getting full credit for the iron that you do consume.

As with other nutrients, too much iron can be dangerous; and we advise caution in taking a supplement as it is intended to be taken. All vitamins containing iron are required to have a childproof cap, because iron in excess can actually be fatal. That is, of course, true only for very large doses. However, a small subset of the population has a condition called hemochromatosis. These people cannot handle even minimal doses of excess iron because it accumulates in their bodies. It then deposits in different organs and can cause liver damage or diabetes, among other issues. Hemochromatosis is a genetic disorder that can be tested for. It is rare but illustrates to us how too much of any substance in the body can ultimately cause harm.

For these reasons, finding the proper iron source in the correct amount is essential. It is also important to find the right means of absorbing that iron to feel more energetic and less fatigued. Iron replacement done right will build back levels over a few months' time and energy can return.

VITAMIN D

The role of vitamin D in general wellness and fatigue has been recently touted. Over the years, we have seen in our practices case after case of patients who feel better once they have optimal levels of vitamin D. The challenge is sticking with taking the vitamin long enough to see its effects. Because it is a fat-soluble vitamin, it often takes six to twelve months to build up circulating blood levels. This means taking it day in and day out to slowly let it accumulate in the body's stores is important. However, once vitamin D levels normalize it is remarkable how much better people feel.

Vitamin D deficiency is an epidemic. The most common way we obtain it is through sunlight. Through the common use of sunscreen (for good reason—preventing skin cancer is so important!), we have minimized our sun exposure. Likewise many people do not get sun because they live in climates where year-round sun exposure is scarce; they spend most of their days indoors; or they are dark skinned and their natural skin color actually prevents vitamin D from penetrating it. Very few natural food sources provide us with vitamin D (the main ones are cow liver or wild-caught salmon—farm raised does not count). A few foods are fortified with D, such as milk and some orange juices, but the amounts are trivial. The majority of us need at least 800 to 1,000 IUs of supplemental vitamin D3 (its most active form—important, because many supplements contain other forms) to maintain a normal blood level.

Determining how much vitamin D you need depends on a variety of factors. Where you live, your skin color, and any conditions that may interfere with vitamin D absorption (such as IBD, celiac, etc.) are important determinants. Blood testing can determine your level. Over decades of seeing thousands of patients, we have found that blood testing is helpful, but rarely mandatory. The majority of our patients are vitamin D deficient unless they are taking a supplement, and the amount needed to correct their deficiency can usually be determined based on the aforementioned factors—diet, preexisting conditions, medications, and current supplement type and amount. When in doubt, D is key.

Future chapters will discuss vitamin D's role in many other areas (bones, cancer prevention, and dementia, among other things). We cannot emphasize enough the importance of this vitamin in maintaining your ideal health. Its role in bone health is incomparable, and it seems to be involved in cellular function in many parts of the body. Therefore, it makes sense that you feel fatigued when you lack vitamin D. It takes months to years to build up your levels, but when you do, its effect is noticeable and important.

VITAMIN B

B vitamins also play a vital role in energy. There are many of them: the obvious ones—B1, B2, B6, B12, as well as some that go by other names, such as thiamine, biotin, folate, riboflavin, and niacin. (You can find out more about each of them in our Vitamin Glossary at the end of the book). The ones that we believe are most essential for maintaining optimal energy levels are vitamins B1 and B12. These vitamins both play important roles in nerve functioning. They help our nerve cells fire smoothly and rapidly. If we lack these vital components, our nerves are essentially sluggish. We then feel these effects as fatigue or sometimes as specific nerve-related symptoms (more on this in later chapters).

The bottom line is B vitamins can be important. We get them from many common food sources (meat, dairy, and some grains and legumes). However, depending on your exact diet and your ability to absorb these vitamins (some people do not absorb certain B vitamins readily because of GI conditions, previous GI surgeries, autoimmune conditions, or medicines that interfere with absorption), you may need some extra.

Many people find B vitamins help boost their energy. However, we do caution that certain "energy" products contain levels of B vitamins that exceed recommended values by many hundreds of times. We do not generally think this is either necessary or good. Significant toxicity can occur from overdoing it with any vitamin, and B vitamins are no exception. Overdoing it with B vitamins can cause flushing, skin problems, and in severe cases almost fatal liver damage (we have seen this in our practices). As with anything you ingest, too much is not a good thing.

IODINE

Another vitamin with great cachet in the "Energy Industry" is iodine, which is essential to thyroid health. The thyroid gland is one of the main ways our body regulates energy and metabolism. The thyroid uses iodine to produce its essential hormone, thyroxine. If we are lacking in iodine, the gland cannot do its job. We then become fatigued. Other signs and symptoms of hypothyroidism are weight gain or trouble losing weight, thinning hair or eyebrows, swelling in the legs, constipation, and a change in menstrual periods. If you believe you have hypothyroidism, you should be screened by your doctor for this relatively common condition.

Worldwide, iodine deficiency is the number one cause of goiters and hypothyroidism. In the 1920s, the United States actually started an iodized salt program in an effort to eliminate the risk of goiter and hypothyroidism in higher risk areas. The United Nations Children's Fund (UNICEF) has been spearheading a worldwide iodized salt program since the 1990s. The intake of iodized salt has helped reduce these conditions.

So should we be taking iodine supplements, and if so, how much? The recommended daily allowance of iodine is 150 micrograms (mcg). There are a number of natural sources of iodine in our diets, including dairy products, saltwater fish, shellfish, soymilk, soy sauce, and seaweed (think sushi!). While many Americans receive the recommended level of iodine in their diet, some people, especially those on a low-salt diet, have decreased the amount of iodine that they ingest. If you cook with only kosher or sea salt, you are more likely to be lacking in iodine. Some multivitamins contain the recommended amount of iodine, while most do not contain any at all. Pregnant and nursing women require even more iodine: 220 and 290 mcg daily, respectively.

Given that many multivitamins don't include iodine, an extra supplement is a good thing, right? Not always! Many commonly sold supplements contain 62 milligrams (mg, not micrograms, mcg) of iodine or more. So that is hundreds of times the recommended amount! That amount of iodine could actually cause hyperthyroidism! Too much iodine can cause your thyroid to "flare up," leading to palpitations and anxiety. It could even lead to heart arrhythmias and osteoporosis, among other serious medical conditions.

MAGNESIUM

We could not complete a discussion about fatigue and energy without mentioning magnesium. This wonderful electrolyte is essential to just about every aspect of our bodily functions. It is the gateway to our cells doing their jobs. For example, muscle cells (including the heart) use magnesium to perform their tasks and feed energy at a cellular level. Not surprisingly then, being low on magnesium can cause all sorts of problems.

Magnesium is found in many common foods, including spinach, legumes, and nuts (see Vitamin Glossary).

However, many of us do not have enough circulating magnesium. Even if we take in a lot of it, we lose it through sweat and other bodily losses. For this reason, we believe that magnesium supplements (in those who do not have kidney disease and have trouble balancing it) can play a very useful role in helping to maintain your energy. They are particularly helpful if you exercise and lose valuable electrolytes, because magnesium also helps the body hold onto potassium (another electrolyte important to cellular function).

———— ◆ ————

Medical causes such as a low thyroid (see more on thyroid disorders in later chapters), anemia, and other endocrine or cardiac abnormalities can all cause fatigue or a lack of energy. See your doctor to rule these out.

Clearly, there is no single answer to improving energy for everyone. Hopefully, you can look at your lifestyle, diet, and health factors to determine which of the discussed tactics can help you feel your very best. Recognize that none of these interventions takes effect immediately. Small changes, maintained over time, are the answer to improving your health. It is sometimes only after months of doing the right things that you can look back and say, "Wow, I really do feel better than I did a few months ago."

CHAPTER 5
VITAMINS FOR HEADACHES— MIGRAINES AND MORE

A VITAMIN A DAY may help keep the doctor away—and it's not that we have anything against your doctor—but many people who suffer from headaches might feel better and have less frequent episodes if they get adequate amounts of the right vitamins. There are actually many different types of headaches. The most common ones are migraines and tension headaches. Migraines are something we see more in our practices, but many people also suffer from low-grade tension headaches for which they don't often seek medical attention. In addition to these varieties of headaches, we will also touch on headaches related to dehydration and other lifestyle factors, such as alcohol (known in medical terms as the hangover).

Migraine Headaches

For those of you who are blessed not to know what a migraine is, it's a type of headache that occurs when blood vessels in the brain spasm. This tends to cause an intense and throbbing headache, often accompanied by nausea, sensitivity to light, or strange visual symptoms. (Please see your doctor to evaluate any symptoms you may have and to confirm your diagnosis.) The most typical location for a migraine is one side of the head, starting behind the eye. However, many people experience pain that involves other parts of their head or their whole head.

Migraines can be debilitating—they can account for significant loss of work time and severely impact a person's quality of life—but they are also common, affecting about 28 million, or 12 percent of Americans. Migraines are in fact more common than asthma and diabetes combined.

Some migraines are accompanied by what is called an "aura," a sensory phenomenon, usually a visual experience (seeing jagged lines, flashes of light, bright spots, or blind spots), that can happen before, during, or after the headache. On rare occasions, these symptoms can occur without an accompanying headache and are then termed a "visual migraine." Some people get auras they describe as a "funny feeling" but can't articulate further.

WHAT TRIGGERS MIGRAINES?

Many, but not all, people who get migraines have a family history of migraines. They can start early in life or come on later. It is rare to develop migraines in later adulthood. Different people have different events or foods that tend to trigger their migraines. It is very common for women to get migraines prior to getting their period (known as a "menstrual migraine"). Other common triggers include changes in weather or barometric pressure, stress, fatigue, or lack of sleep. In addition, many foods and food additives are known to trigger migraines in certain people. The most common culprits include red wine, chocolate, aged cheeses, nitrates, and monosodium glutamate (MSG).

So what's a migraine sufferer to do? Firstly, avoid trigger foods when at all possible (especially in those days prior to your period). Also be sure to stay well-hydrated with water and adequate electrolytes. Regular sleep is also important, of course. (Heard that one before? We seem to harp on it a lot, but that's only because it's tied to so many aspects of health.)

Another factor to consider in the migraine equation is caffeine, which is actually useful in treating or aborting migraines for many sufferers. In fact, many over-the-counter migraine treatments (such as Excedrin Migraine) include common pain medications combined with caffeine. The flip side of this positive effect of caffeine is the withdrawal phenomenon. Regular caffeine use followed by abruptly stopping caffeine intake is a classic trigger for a migraine. The solution: Stay consistent in your caffeine use and wean down if you want to cut back. Cutting off caffeine cold turkey can be unpleasant in many ways, migraine included.

Another rebound issue can occur with over-the-counter pain meds. Specifically, ibuprofen products or what we call NSAIDs (nonsteriodal anti-inflammatory drugs, which include common brands such as Aleve, Motrin, and Advil) can cause withdrawal headaches if used with regularity. People who take these products continually get caught in a vicious cycle. Eventually they get headaches as the drugs wear off, so they feel compelled to keep taking the medicine. Therefore, it is best to avoid using these drugs daily. If you already do so, you should wean off them gradually to minimize rebound. While weaning and instead of using this type of pain reliever, one can try acetaminophen products, which are less likely to cause rebound issues. Do be cautious to follow package instructions and do not overuse these either.

Treatment for migraines once they occur is a huge topic that is beyond the scope of this book. Needless to say, there are many, many treatments for acute migraine. In addition, a number of drugs for daily prevention or "prophylaxis" of migraines are available for those who suffer from frequent headaches of this type. The decision about what treatment is best for you is an individual choice to discuss with your doctor.

However, before you take prescription medication for migraine prevention, you may want to first consider some vitamin solutions that have been proven helpful at reducing migraine frequency.

MAGNESIUM FOR MIGRAINES

We are big believers in magnesium for its role in migraine prevention (as well as many other health issues—see the Constipation, Immunity and Body Aches, Bone Health, and Blood Pressure chapters in this book). Magnesium is a vital electrolyte that we get from many natural foods (namely, low levels are found in nuts, beans, spinach, and a variety of grains). Cells and systems all over our body need it to function properly (including those blood vessels in your brain). Our kidneys regulate magnesium, potassium, and other electrolytes in a complicated balance.

Many of us walk around with suboptimal blood levels of magnesium, in part because most food sources contain very low levels of the vitamin. Also, we continually lose magnesium through many normal body functions and even through exercise (via muscle use and sweat).

While there is certainly still more to learn about the role of electrolytes in migraine treatments, new data suggests that replacing magnesium may help prevent and treat migraines. We can assume this is true because of this essential nutrient's role in making blood vessels function optimally, but the exact science is not yet fully understood. No matter the precise reason magnesium helps, it does in fact help. Several large studies have shown it reduces the frequency of migraines in those who get them. For this reason it is probably a helpful electrolyte to take.

A typical dose for migraine prevention is 300 or 400 mg daily. Most of our patients tolerate this dose well without any side effects. However, higher doses of magnesium are known to cause GI side effects such as cramping and diarrhea. If you stick to this dose, most people are fine. Another thing to be aware of is that your kidneys can only handle so much of this stuff, and if you have kidney disease you should for sure limit your intake. However, if you are an otherwise healthy person, magnesium supplementation, when taken in safe doses, may be a great step in helping you kiss those migraines goodbye.

B VITAMINS FOR MIGRAINES

Another vitamin that has come into favor since 2010 for migraine prevention is vitamin B2 or riboflavin. This vitamin is found in small amounts in natural foods such as meat, cheese, eggs, and nuts. However, those who suffer from migraines may benefit from supplementation. A dose of 400 mg daily of B2 has been shown to reduce the frequency of migraines. The role of other B vitamins in migraine prevention and treatment is less established. It is known that vitamin

B12 plays a role in many neurological issues, but it has not been definitively shown that taking it prevents or treats migraines.

VITAMIN D

Vitamin D has been researched for migraine prevention. However, the data thus far is not compelling for migraines, though it may be useful for preventing other types of headaches (such as tension headaches, which are dull headaches without associated symptoms, typically occurring at the end of the day). Nonetheless, we are big fans of vitamin D for its many other proven benefits. (See the Bone Health and Immunity and Body Aches chapters in this book, among others.)

VITAMIN COQ10

CoQ10 is another vitamin that has been suggested to be helpful for migraine sufferers. A few studies have shown that it may be effective in migraine prevention at doses of up to 100 mg three times daily. The potential side effects are unknown. At the time of this writing, we believe CoQ10 is an intriguing possible prevention for migraine, but the data is less proven than that of other vitamins. Therefore, it should be used only after other options have failed.

———— ◆ ————

All in all, we believe vitamins can play an important role in migraine prevention. If you have a verified history of migraines, starting a vitamin regimen tailored to their prevention can be a great help. There are of course many prescription treatments that, if needed, you can discuss with your physician. In addition, any increasing or changes in your symptoms should be brought to his or her attention. However, it is our hope that if you employ some of the lifestyle and vitamin strategies we have discussed, your migraines will be a thing of the past.

Tension Headaches

Tension headaches are aptly named as they result from a tensing of the muscles around the head. They are typically brought on by stress, or sometimes dehydration. They are often described as a band-like sensation around the head, and they tend to occur later in the day. They are not typically associated with symptoms like nausea, vomiting, visual changes, or sensitivity to light.

Of course, any new symptoms or changes in headache pattern warrant evaluation by a physician.

Tension headaches are often successfully treated with simple over-the-counter analgesics or pain relievers such as acetaminophen or ibuprofen. Sometimes the addition of caffeine can be helpful, though less so than in migraine treatment. The perils of daily use of these medications is of course the potential for a "rebound effect," which may occur more often in headaches of the tension type. Daily use of any over-the-counter medication should be avoided for this reason and because ibuprofen-type medications often can cause GI side effects such as ulcers.

As with many chronic conditions, tension headaches can be reduced in frequency and severity with some lifestyle adjustments. Not surprisingly, sleep can be important. (More on sleep habits and hygiene in our Sleep chapter.) In addition, stress relievers can be very useful for tension headache relief. For each person, this may be something different. It may mean a change in daily work schedule or more frequent breaks. For some, it may mean learning yoga, meditation practices, or a medical treatment called cognitive behavioral therapy, which teaches relaxation techniques via some physical cues. For others, stress reduction may mean quitting your job, sending your kids to boarding school, asking your spouse to have a lobotomy, and kicking back with friends and a bottle of wine.

Headaches Related to Dehydration

To relieve tension headaches and many other types of headaches, hydration is essential. One commonly overlooked element when it comes to hydration is the importance of electrolytes. When we see patients and suggest lack of hydration is contributing to a condition, they often pull out their trusty water bottle and say, "I drink all day long." While water is of course essential, "free water" (meaning water without any electrolytes) is often not enough to stay hydrated. The body uses electrolytes in the blood stream to actually hold onto the water (if you think way back to high school chemistry and osmosis, you may recall that water goes where the ions are). Therefore, essential electrolytes, such as sodium, potassium, and chloride, are important for staying hydrated. Magnesium is also important since it is involved in how your kidneys balance all the others.

For this reason, we advise our patients not to drink only water. Electrolyte replacement via either food sources or beverages is important. This is particularly true when discussing headaches. Many people report worse headaches when their "blood sugar is low." These cases are actually rarely due to a true low blood sugar (this only happens in people who take medication for diabetes or have a rare form of pancreatic tumor), but in fact are due to drops in many of the other vital ingredients that come from eating and drinking enough. Some people are particularly sensitive to not eating regularly and should work hard to keep hydrated and consume sufficient electrolytes by eating frequent small meals and taking in electrolyte-rich fluids. These can be in the form of juices or sports drinks (mixing them with water can cut down on the excess sugar while still providing the essential electrolytes.). Thus the "low blood sugar" sensation is actually a real feeling that is telling you that you are missing important nutrients. These can be electrolytes or just plain energy, which can also be obtained from good protein or fat sources (more on this in the Nutrition chapter).

A normal person's blood sugar can drop to a low normal value just from eating the typical American breakfast of cereal with milk, orange juice, and toast. The high carb and sugar load leads blood sugars to plummet midmorning after digestion is completed. Adding some fats and protein to complex carbs, via eggs or peanut butter with your whole wheat toast for instance, can help sustain you for longer.

During the day, it never hurts to have a quick snack. A jar of peanut butter in your desk is useful to have on hand. Yogurt, low-fat cheese, or nuts are other healthful snacks.

At Vous Vitamin®, we created our Power Up Situational Supplement™ expressly for the purpose of replenishing lost electrolytes. It provides essential electrolytes and B vitamins in tablet form. It is recommended to be taken with a large glass of water several times daily when you are exercising or having an intense day. It helps keep your body going by providing these nutrients that we often lose when we sweat or work hard. Power Up™ does not have any calories, sugar, or caffeine. Beware of other "energy" products that do and can cause a "high" sensation followed by a "crash," leaving your energy feeling more depleted than before.

Headaches Related to Alcohol

Clearly hydration with water and nutrients is essential for headache treatment and prevention. Another instance where this comes into play is when alcohol is involved. Few of us have escaped adult life without paying for an evening out on the town. As we get beyond our twenties, many of us have found it sometimes doesn't seem worth it to enjoy a drink or two because it tends to wreak havoc on our night's sleep and the next day.

We are not necessarily pushing abstinence here. Rather, we think moderation is key. One can also employ some techniques to avoid headaches related to alcohol and the dreaded hangover. Turns out much of alcohol's ill effects come from its tendency to dehydrate you and specifically your brain cells. Alcohol has a well-known diuretic effect (witness any bathroom line at a big event for proof). Excessive urination quickly saps both your body and your brain of fluids. Your brain gets particularly testy about this, and you feel it big time.

The above principles of consuming lots of water and the proper electrolytes can help in this area as well. There are also a few key vitamins that come into play when alcohol is involved. We learned in medical school that when anyone shows up in the emergency room intoxicated, the first thing that happens is they hang an IV bag full of bright yellow solution, referred to as a "banana bag." This concoction, which frankly looks a lot like urine, is not only important in replacing important vitamins and electrolytes, but it also holds the cure to the common hangover. It's chock-full of thiamine (vitamin B1), folic acid, and magnesium, and these help compete with alcohol to block certain receptors in the brain and combat the effects of dehydration.

We can't all hook up an IV every time we have a cocktail (though there are actually some companies out there doing this, for a hefty fee!). We can, however, work on ways to keep our own brain cells nice and hydrated as well as full of the right vitamins. At Vous Vitamin®, we created our Recovery Act Situation Supplement™ for this purpose. These little yellow pills are essentially a banana bag you can keep in your pocket. Take one with some water while drinking and again in the morning, and many of our customers say they are in great shape the next day. Anyone who suffers from headaches related to alcohol consumption can try this combination with plenty of water. You can certainly skip the cocktails all together, but that can put a bit of a damper on your night out.

———————— ♦ ————————

Headaches of the migraine variety or other types can be an unpleasant part of life. Each type of headache can often be averted with certain lifestyle interventions, such as regular sleep, balanced eating, and hydration. Certain headaches are amenable to vitamins as a part of treatment and prevention and can be used in addition to numerous medical therapies.

CHAPTER 6
VITAMINS FOR THINNING HAIR

AS A PRIMARY CARE PHYSICIAN and an endocrinologist, there is one concern we both hear all the time from men and women alike—thinning hair. This complaint is both distressing and common. While men and women both express concerns, the reason for their hair loss can be different, but sometimes the root cause is the same (pun intended). Some hair loss is inevitable with age, but there are some easily reversible causes to this vexing problem, and vitamins are often a part of the solution.

Hair loss for men is a commonly discussed topic. It is, in fact, a billion-dollar industry, flush with over-the-counter products, pharmaceuticals, transplantation procedures, and more. Yet we don't even have a Hair Club for Women. But we should.

Hair loss and hair thinning is, in fact, a very common complaint of women of all ages. As physicians, hair loss in women is something we hear about daily. Yes, you heard us correctly. We have joked that a day at the office is not complete without some woman crying over her hair thinning, but it is in fact no laughing matter. This problem is a cause of great distress, and it should be taken very seriously. It seems that many women fear that it is a permanent state of affairs. However, our experience tells us it can most often be reversed or improved.

A substantial part of male hair loss is hormonal. What is described in the medical world as male pattern baldness is the typical receding hairline men get as they age and bald. The hairline above their forehead starts to slowly creep back. Sometimes it is cleverly disguised with a combover or other stealthy techniques. The crown can also start to thin out. These days, many men seem to go for broke and just shave their whole head at the sign of recession. We love the spirit of cutting your losses and going all out with the shave, but we caution that some men may be a bit hasty with this strategy, since there may in fact be options to help keep your head of hair intact.

Male pattern baldness is caused by testosterone, the most male of hormones. All men have testosterone, but certain men seem to produce higher levels at older ages and a more active form that leads to the previously described pattern of loss. What can be done? To address the hormonal issue, a number of both topical and oral medications exist (which you can discuss with your doctor). These typically serve the same purpose: They act by blocking the testosterone receptors so the hormone does not take its toll. Propecia® is a prescription oral drug. Topical agents like minoxidil (also known by the brand name Rogaine®) block the effects of testosterone on the hair follicles locally. They can be helpful, but they only work as long as you keep applying them and they tend not to cause any regrowth of lost hair. Rather, they help maintain what hair you have. For men, this is particularly helpful if they start early. However, once you stop these medicines, the hair you tried to maintain tends to fall out. There are concerns that these drugs can contribute to male infertility, and some men note side effects such as sexual dysfunction, which should come as no surprise, given the drugs' testosterone-blocking effects. In addition, because of these products' effects on testosterone in male fetuses, women of childbearing age should not use them and pregnant women should not even touch them.

While the majority of women suffer from a diffuse thinning of the hair, some women actually suffer from male pattern baldness, which involves a generalized thinning of the hair and a recession at the temples and crown. Since the whole-head shave is not typically considered a great option for women, we must look to other solutions. One is a prescription medication called spironolactone (or Aldactone®, its brand name). This medicine is used for a number of medical conditions including heart and liver failure, but happens to also block testosterone receptors. It can be prescribed to women for male pattern baldness, with some success, although women who are pregnant or planning to be pregnant soon should not use it. In fact, they should be on birth control if pregnancy is a possibility. The use of Aldactone® also requires monitoring of electrolytes. It also takes many months to take effect, so patience is a must. This is a decision to discuss with your physician.

Other solutions for men or women include hair transplantation, a process that has come a long way in the 2000s and if done by an experienced practitioner can be a great solution for those with severe male pattern baldness.

Other types of baldness should also be considered. For example, alopecia areata is an autoimmune condition where a limited area of hair falls out, leaving a big bald patch. This can be treated by a dermatologist, often with topical steroids. Another condition is called trichotillomania and is characterized by a compulsion to pull out one's own hair. It can mimic alopecia areata in that bald patches arise, but they are self-inflicted. This is a psychiatric problem and should be addressed by a trained mental health professional.

Hair loss or thinning can occur in association with mental or physical stress, pregnancy (for up to two years following delivery), hormone imbalances (especially thyroid issues and occasionally after stopping birth control), autoimmune disorders, in association with certain medications (and over-the-counter supplements—specifically, DHEA supplements marketed for "adrenal fatigue"), or occasionally after stopping birth control pills.

If the above conditions are not present, we are left with what we most typically see as a cause for hair loss or diffuse thinning of the hair, vitamin deficiencies, which thankfully is a correctable problem. Certain nutrients are vital for healthy hair. Correcting deficiencies takes some time and patience, but it *can* help with hair loss!

The vitamins and minerals most women lack for proper hair health are vitamin D and iron. We commonly see women (and men) who do not and cannot get enough of either of these important nutrients in their diet. Women lose iron through menstruation and pregnancy.

Also, we no longer live in a carnivorous society where we scarf down red meat at multiple meals a day.

While eating less meat may be great for other health and environmental or humane reasons, it is not so helpful when it comes to maintaining appropriate levels of iron. As a result, eventually we see signs of iron depletion in the form of hair loss, fatigue, and other symptoms. If you are experiencing any of these symptoms, the first step is to consult with your doctor as these symptoms may be signs of something more serious. Sometimes, additional testing is warranted. Typical blood testing (a blood count) may not reveal these deficiencies since despite whole body stores being low, the blood count can still appear normal.

Specific lab testing for ferritin or iron stores can be helpful. However, it is our experience that most women complaining of hair loss are iron depleted. Through a plan of gradual replacement (in the correct combination with other nutrients that help with iron absorption, such as vitamin C), this problem can be fixed. But it does not happen overnight. It takes six to twelve months. Typically a ferritin level needs to be built up to over 70 nanograms per milliliter in order to see hair regrowth, even though the lab's normal may be 11 or above. Patience with this issue is difficult, but we are sure that every woman who has done it would tell you, it is well worth the wait.

Similarly, a vitamin D deficiency is a very common contributor to the hair loss dilemma. Vitamin D is an important vitamin that plays a vital role in bone metabolism, immunity, and many other physiological processes. Getting enough vitamin D strictly through our diet (mostly found in wild-caught salmon or beef liver) is very challenging. While the sun gives us vitamin D, we all know by now that excess exposure to the sun can cause skin cancer and other ailments. Thus, sunbathing is most definitely not recommended as a source for our vitamin D. People who live in more temperate climates do not generally have enough sun exposure year-round to keep their vitamin D stores up. Additionally, our kidneys and liver must convert the metabolite we obtain from the sun into its active form and our bodies do not often process the vitamin D as they should.

Fear not, vitamin D also is a nutrient that we can replenish over time. Like iron, it requires a steady daily dose over many months, and the amount taken should not be excessive (too much of a good thing is not better, but can in fact be harmful). It also is best taken in its most active form, vitamin D3. Restoring appropriate levels of vitamin D should enable you to restore your body to its optimal level of function.

Hair growth would not be stimulated without providing your body with its natural building blocks. For this we turn to biotin, another nutrient that plays an essential role in nail and hair growth, in the latter case, specifically the repair and regrowth of hair follicles. Biotin dosing varies greatly, but most dermatologists who specialize in hair loss believe a dose of 2,500 mcg daily is appropriate. It of course takes time to see the effects (you should be used to hearing that by now).

With time and the consistent use of vitamins, hair loss related to deficiencies slowly improves. At Vous Vitamin®, we have found that thinning hair is one of the most common complaints expressed by our customers on our online questionnaire. Our multivitamins (with a blend of the aforementioned vitamins) that address this issue are some of our top sellers. We have found that if people are patient and diligent about taking their vitamins, they find their hair returns to a better state. Many men say that even though their male pattern of balding does not resolve, the thickness and growth of their existing hair improves with vitamin repletion and they feel that it enhances their feeling of a fuller head of hair.

The distressing issue of hair loss never has a quick and easy fix. However, with some exploration and diligence there are many ways to address it. We find vitamins are often a key part of the solution.

CHAPTER 7
ANXIETY AND DEPRESSION

HAILEY IS A PATIENT who came into Arielle's office and burst into tears. "I'm a mess!" she said. "I yell at my kids all the time, my husband thinks I'm crazy, and I wake up every night worrying about the littlest things. I feel terrible every day, like I don't have the energy to get anything done. What is wrong with me?"

Feeling like a nervous wreck? Up at night with to-do lists and worry lists running through your head? Or perhaps the opposite: lying in bed, having trouble finding the motivation or inspiration to get up and do anything? Feeling like the daily grind is too much to handle sometimes? Edgy and emotional to the point that you commonly snap at family members or coworkers?

These symptoms of anxiety and/or depression are some of the most common we hear about in our practices. It is of course very common for many people to have times in their lives when they feel particularly anxious or down in the dumps and depressed. There is a range in severity of these symptoms and accordingly there is a range in the type of treatment needed to address them. This is by no means an attempt to provide a comprehensive approach to mental health issues; rather, it is a discussion of how vitamins may be a part of that conversation. However, to contextualize vitamins' role properly, let's first discuss how anxiety and depression are typically treated in the United States today.

It goes without saying that severe forms of anxiety and depression, and any indication of wanting to harm oneself or others, are matters that should be addressed by a qualified health-care professional. This chapter focuses not on these more urgent interventions, but on ways in which vitamins may play a role in treating some of these symptoms, either as stand-alone solutions or, more often, as a part of a comprehensive plan that may include prescription medication, lifestyle interventions, and a therapy component.

Anxiety and depression so often go hand in hand. While in some ways these conditions' symptoms represent opposite ends of the spectrum (anxiety = more wired and hyper; depressed = more lethargic and low energy), there is still a great deal of overlap. In other words, many people experience both either simultaneously or intermittently; therefore, the treatments also have some overlap and some distinctions. Many prescription medications are coindicated for both anxiety and depression, while others are not. Likewise, many supplements have been recommended for use in both conditions, but some are more specific to those with anxiety-type symptoms, while others are more geared toward depression. In our discussion, we will talk about both anxiety and depression separately and will include the different vitamins useful for each condition. There is some overlap, but we feel it's important to discuss each vitamin as it relates to the specific symptoms.

First, let's explore anxiety. It is a disorder with a huge spectrum of manifestations. This state of feeling unsettled, nervous, and overly concerned can often be accompanied by very physical manifestations. Many people experience chronic low levels of anxiety that underlie their daily lives, while others experience very discrete episodes of full-scale panic attacks with extremely physical symptoms, such as a sensation of palpitations, chest discomfort, or trouble breathing. Needless to say, you should consult with your health-care provider about any of these complaints, since some other medical conditions can cause similar symptoms. If anxiety is in fact determined to be the cause, then there are a number of approaches to consider.

There are lifestyle interventions that can be useful. Getting regular exercise is a wonderful way to blow off steam and help reduce anxiety. During exercise your body senses that it is time to release certain stress hormones and endorphins. These are the hormones that help raise your heart rate and blood pressure and get your mind hyper-focused. This is a strikingly similar experience to a moment of anxiety or panic. With exercise, however, when you stop the activity, the body gradually returns to normal. Doing this on a regular basis keeps your body trained to go through this ritual when exercising, but not so much at other times. Regular exercise actually lowers your resting heart rate between exercise episodes. It has been reported that superstar athletes like Michael Jordan have resting heart rates in the 30s (normal for adults is typically 60–90). Sometimes just taking a vigorous walk can go a long way toward melting away anxiety. Even better if it's with a friend and you can talk it out a bit!

Beyond cardio exercise, a multitude of other regular habits can be extremely effective in minimizing anxiety. Disciplines in mindfulness and meditation as well as yoga and Pilates are all means to learn breathing techniques and mental strategies that help your body naturally calm itself. These disciplines bear striking similarity to techniques of cognitive behavioral therapy, which teaches practitioners to use their own physical cues and body awareness to promote self-regulated techniques for reducing stress and anxiety. Guided imagery techniques for meditation can accomplish similar results. These are worthwhile pursuits for anyone with anxiety of any type and seem especially helpful for those with situational anxiety (i.e., anxiety triggered in certain predictable situations such as a fear of flying, heights, etc.).

A discussion of prescription medication is well beyond this the scope of this book, but should be considered under the guidance of a professional. One important thing to understand about medication for anxiety is that there are two distinct, but not mutually exclusive options—daily medication and as-needed-type medications. There are several commonly used classes of daily medications for depression: serotonin-specific reuptake inhibitors (SSRIs), serotonin-norepinephrine reuptake inhibitors (SNRIs), and a few others. These are medications that are taken regularly with the hope of preventing symptoms of anxiety (or depression). They can be wonderful, if not life-changing treatment for many people, but often require some trial and error to find the right fit for each individual. They also take some time to stop and start—that is, they take several weeks if not months to build up in your system to be effective. On the back end, they generally require a weaning period to stop them to avoid nasty withdrawal symptoms. In addition, taking daily medication is a commitment, as one should take it for at least six to twelve months.

Medication is certainly not for everyone. However, one common issue we see in practice is that people who are anxiety ridden and may benefit from medication the most are so anxious about taking medication that they do not give it a try. If your health professional recommends that you consider daily medication for a psychiatric concern, you should be open to the option and hold some trust in your provider's ability to choose a medication that is likely to help your situation. This is a bit of a leap of faith when you are feeling overly concerned about everything around you, but it is sometimes worth that extra push to try something. Staring at a bottle of medication for weeks on end and pondering whether to take it is not going to help your situation at all. Taking action may.

In addition to daily medications, there are as-needed medication options for anxiety (which unfortunately are less useful for depression). These typically are medicine in the class of benzodiazepines or valium-type medications. They work quickly (within minutes) and effectively to minimize anxiety symptoms and last several hours or more. However, they have some major limitations—primarily that they are a quick fix and do not really treat the underlying symptoms. Thus those symptoms can quickly return once the drug wears off. These valium-like medications are also sedating, often impairing one's ability to function. They should not be taken before driving. Another important concern is that they are habit-forming. Over time you may need to take more and more of the medication to get the desired effect. You may also experience serious withdrawal if you stop them abruptly. In our opinion, there is a limited role for these medications—they should be used only occasionally for extreme circumstances or for very specific anxiety-inducing situations such as fear of flying or heights. They are rarely a long-term solution to anxiety.

The effects of prescription medications may be augmented with certain vitamins, or vitamins may even be part of a solution to avoid medication when possible. Some of the most common vitamins recommended for anxiety and depression have considerable scientific data to back their use, while others have less. Our firsthand experiences have guided our recommendations for a few worth trying.

Anxiety, not surprisingly, can be treated with some of the same supplements discussed for aiding with sleep. Both processes involve a reduction of agitation and a relaxation component. Some supplements have been touted for working on various neurotransmitters to ·stimulate relaxation. These include valerian root, kava, chamomile, and gamma-aminobutyric acid (GABA). All are said to bind to the receptors centered in the relaxation areas of the brain. As with many herbal supplements, the data is somewhat lacking. While some people do find success with these products, it is our experience that most do not see noticeable improvements from using them. In addition, they can present issues with purity and contamination by other unintended ingredients. Vous Vitamin® has not felt comfortable manufacturing or endorsing these particular products because we do not see enough evidence in their favor. If you do feel strongly about trying some of these products, we recommend using only well-made ones from reputable sources.

The other types of vitamins often touted for anxiety are those with anti-inflammatory properties. These include the omega-3s (typically as fish oil) and vitamin C. Both have some decent evidence to suggest that they can be helpful for anxiety. Exactly why inflammation is part of the problem remains unclear. However, given that both omega-3s and vitamin C are generally safe in moderate doses (we believe no more than 2,000 mg of the first and 500 mg of the latter), they are worth considering. We make reference to many of their other health benefits in other chapters of this book (e.g., Cholesterol, and Immunity and Body Aches).

Some other vitamins that might diminish anxiety are vitamin B12 and folic acid. Both of these B vitamins seem to have important roles in nerve function. They may make our nerves function more optimally since their deficiencies lead to a variety of disturbances in the nervous system. It makes sense that replacing them in someone experiencing symptoms of anxiety may be helpful.

The other vitamin that is likely to play an important role in easing anxiety symptoms is magnesium. This essential nutrient plays a key role in optimal cellular function, as it regulates various channels that then allow cells to perform as they should. This seems to aid in reducing anxiety and its physical symptoms. We also discuss magnesium in our Sleep chapter, as, not surprisingly, it helps with sleep as well. It is our finding that daily magnesium supplementation is more useful than occasional as-needed use. At Vous Vitamin®, magnesium is a common component of many of our Personalized Multivitamins™.

While anxiety symptoms can be treated and prevented using a number of vitamins, depression can also be alleviated by several vitamins and supplements. The role of prescription medication in treating depression is similar to anxiety though some of the actual agents' uses vary slightly. The concept of daily medication should be discussed with your health-care provider. Additionally psychotherapy should also be considered, either individually or in a group setting, since many studies and our experience shows that medication and therapy in combination tend to be more effective than either alone. Vitamins can often be used to enhance these modalities or, for some people, as a remedy for mild symptoms.

One key vitamin that can play a part in depression is vitamin D. In fact, we have seen many patients with vitamin D deficiency who felt depressed and felt their symptoms were much improved with repletion of this nutrient. It is interesting that one source of vitamin D is the sun and many people suffer from Seasonal Affective Disorder, a condition where they become more depressed during winter months. Replacing vitamin D should therefore be a year-round affair. The fat-soluble nature of this vitamin makes it slow to build up levels, and it's important to maintain them with supplemental D in preparation for the winter months. That is because it must make its way into fat and remain stored there. In 2015 some evidence was found to suggest a link between vitamin D and serotonin production. Serotonin is the mood-enhancing neurotransmitter that many antidepressants aim to increase. (For more information on vitamin D and its sources, see the Thinning Hair chapter and the Vitamin Glossary.)

Vitamin B12 and folic acid may be useful in the treatment of depression. We previously discussed their role in reducing anxiety, and there seems to be good data to suggest an association with low levels of these B vitamins and depression. Thus, correcting them only makes sense. Another B vitamin, B1 or thiamine, is also known to play a role in the nervous system, and its deficiency is also associated with symptoms that can mimic depression.

When speaking of depression, another often talked about supplement is St. John's wort. This plant-derived herb has been touted for its miraculous mood-boosting effects. However, the data is not so compelling, nor is our clinical experience. Rather, we have seen its dangerous effects (often when combined with other medications such as traditional antidepressants and migraine therapies). St. John's wort can cause serotonin syndrome (see the Vitamin Horror Stories in chapter 3), and we have seen numerous cases of liver function abnormality when people take this type of supplement alone or in combination with other medications. We do not find this supplement worth the effort or the potential risks when looking to aid those suffering from depression.

Omega-3s, which may help with anxiety, might also play an important role in depression, though precisely why they help remains unknown (perhaps the anti-inflammatory effect). As we've mentioned, these are generally well-tolerated in the form of fish oil or flaxseed oil and can be a useful addition to a vitamin regimen. We advise no more than 2,000 mg daily from a pure and reputable brand. Omega-3s seem to play a role in treating so many inflammation-mediated processes including cardiovascular disease and arthritis. At Vous Vitamin®, they are an important part of our next wave of product development.

————————◆————————

Now back to Hailey, our distressed thirty-one-year-old patient. After a long discussion with her about her current symptoms and her emotional and medical history, it became clear she was suffering from a combination of depressive symptoms and anxiety. Her anxiety was disrupting her sleep, and she was exhausted and irritable by day. It was hard to tell what had come first, but clearly both issues needed to be addressed. Through a combination of lifestyle changes (better diet, regular exercise that for her included yoga and meditation), talk therapy, and some specific vitamin suggestions, her situation improved markedly. She returned several months later to report that she was feeling like a new person, employing a combination of magnesium, vitamin D, and B vitamins seemed to help her sleep and alleviated both her anxiety symptoms and her daytime depression.

All in all there are a number of vitamins and supplements that may be helpful in aiding with symptoms of both anxiety and depression. As with any symptoms, it is important to consider a global approach to each person and how different treatments may fit into their lives. A traditional approach to treating anxiety and depression can include lifestyle optimization such as exercise and possibly meditation, prescription medication, and psychotherapy. A thoughtful vitamin regimen is an important consideration in treatment of anxiety and/or depressive symptoms. Vitamins can complement these other modalities and help act as a preventative. They may be an important addition and a useful tool to minimize these distressing symptoms.

CHAPTER 8
ALL SYSTEMS GO

BATTLING CONSTIPATION AND IRRITABLE BOWEL SYNDROME THE NATURAL WAY

FEELING BACKED UP, bloated, and constipated? Guess what? You are not alone. Constipation is something many people suffer from—young and old. By definition it is somewhat subjective. Meaning, there is no hard-and-fast rule about how often someone should have a bowel movement. For some, their normal is to go every day. For others it is to go a few times a day. The problem arises if you experience GI distress.

The official definition of constipation includes hard stool, straining with defecation, or going less than three times per week. Studies suggest that about 15 percent of people suffer from this problem at any given time. It is more common in women and adults over sixty-five, but can happen to anyone.

If you experience these symptoms, you should of course check with your own doctor to rule out underlying problems. Warning signs of more serious issues can include a sudden change in your bowel habits, blood in your stool, fever, unexplained weight loss, and persistent abdominal pain. Assuming there are no underlying blockages or medical conditions, you can start to treat the symptoms of chronic constipation, or what can be a form of Irritable Bowel Syndrome (IBS), with vitamins and supplements in conjunction with other healthful habits.

What Is IBS?

This is a term you will hear batted around quite a bit these days. Firstly, IBS should not be confused with IBD, or Inflammatory Bowel Disease (a term for Crohn's disease and ulcerative colitis, which are autoimmune-type conditions, requiring treatment by a gastroenterologist). In contrast, IBS is a less well-defined condition and essentially is a term for GI symptoms (constipation and/or diarrhea, bloating, discomfort) that cannot be attributed to another cause. If all testing is negative for things like IBD, cancers, infections, and celiac sprue (a serious intolerance to gluten), then symptoms are attributed to IBS. As you can imagine, this means there are many different varieties of IBS out there.

For the purpose of this writing, we will focus predominantly on constipation and mixed IBS (characterized by both diarrhea and constipation). The reality is both are treated similarly. That is because they are both due to a dysregulation of the GI tract. In other words, the normal biorhythms that tell your colon when to move things along are out of whack. Essentially your system needs to be retrained. Using the right combination of dietary changes and natural products, this can often be done simply, safely, and effectively.

Let's start with an example: We saw a college student who complained that she was only moving her bowels once per week. Not surprisingly, in the days in between, she felt bloated, uncomfortable, and sluggish. She had on occasion used over-the-counter stimulant laxatives for constipation relief, but felt they were "hard on her system" and worked unpredictably (not so convenient when you are sitting in class!). She would on rare occasions also have unexpected bouts of loose stools, preceded by cramping. She was tired of living with these symptoms and very frustrated that her efforts to alleviate her symptoms seemed to backfire.

The college student with these symptoms needed help in several areas.

First, we had to improve her hydration status. She was not consuming enough fluids every day. We added a regimen of drinking eight ounces (oz.) of water four times daily to her usual routine to aid in her constipation relief.

She also was not exercising in any meaningful way. Believe it or not, getting your whole body moving also helps get your GI tract moving. Luckily it's usually not at the same time!

Once these simple modifications were in place our patient felt better, but she was still troubled by some mild symptoms. At that point, we introduced a high-fiber diet for additional constipation relief. Some great dietary sources of fiber include prunes, apples, pears, raisins, grapes, and legumes. Our patient started eating oat bran daily for breakfast and when unable to take in 25 grams of fiber per day, she supplemented with a fiber powder (we recommend supplemental fiber such as methylcellulose or psyllium fiber supplements such as Benefiber® or Citrucel® powders, not capsules, with lots of water!). For maintenance, a constipation relief regimen can also include crushed flaxseed (not whole) such as Bob's Red Mill®, two tablespoons twice daily sprinkled in food (delicious in yogurt or a salad, unnoticeable in baked goods).

A diet that is worthy of mention when discussing IBS is the FODMAP diet. A funny sounding constellation of letters, this diet represents an equally bizarre and disparate group of foods to avoid. The theory is that these foods contain certain carbohydrates (specifically the fermentable oligosaccharides, disaccharides, mono-saccharides, and polyols) that cause fermentation in the GI tract, which leads to cramping, bloating, and pain. The list includes garlic, onions, cauliflower, apples, many wheat products, certain artificial sweeteners, and many dairy products, among other things. Certainly this could be very limiting. However, it is worth checking out if you suffer from chronic GI symptoms, since there is data to support its effectiveness in both IBS and IBD (such as Crohn's). Numerous patients of ours have found it very helpful. However, it is not an all-or-nothing proposition; rather it can be used as a guide for what foods might exacerbate symptoms and to try avoiding.

What about Other Over-the-Counter Laxatives?

It is important to know what exactly you are taking here. There is a difference between stool softeners (such as docusate products) and stimulant laxatives. Stool softeners are perfectly safe and can be taken long term without any untoward effects. In fact, they are commonly given during pregnancy and the postpartum period. Stimulant laxatives (such as bisacodyl, senna, or sennoside products) can be effective in the short term, but should not be taken with regularity. They can ultimately cause more harm than good by making your colon dependent on them to work. They are not a long-term solution to constipation or IBS. Conversely, "osmotic laxatives," such as polyethylene glycol (PEG) simply draw fluid into the colon, not stimulating it to contract, and are safe to use daily and chronically.

Is it true that some vitamins can contribute to constipation? Some elemental vitamins such as iron and calcium can be binding and contribute to slowing down the GI tract. One of the most common reasons people stop taking certain vitamins is because of GI issues. However, certain forms of nutrients, such as iron in the form carbonyl and calcium gluconate, are much less likely to cause GI distress. If the proper nutrients are balanced appropriately in the right combination, constipation is much less likely to become a problem. At Vous Vitamin® we work hard to create multivitamin formulations that do not cause GI symptoms given this is such a common cause for people not taking vitamins.

What Vitamins Can Help with Constipation?

In addition to the diet and exercise suggestions, adding some vitamins and minerals also may be helpful in constipation relief. Magnesium is a natural form of a laxative. It helps stimulate your GI tract to operate smoothly. Magnesium channels are essential in making cells cause muscle contractions, and the GI tract is a muscle too! Many of us can benefit from a little more magnesium in our diet. However, too much is never a good thing. Those who have compromised kidney function should stay clear of magnesium-containing products as it can be dangerous for them.

Another vitamin solution to constipation is fish oil or omega-3s. Vous Vitamin® is considering them in our next line of product development, because omega-3s seem to play a role in helping many issues. In regard to GI health, these can often act as natural laxatives, likely because they act as a natural lubricant or stool softener. Most people taking omega-3s are taking them for other reasons (triglyceride lowering or joint health) but notice this beneficial side effect of less constipation. However, for some this can backfire, and omega-3s can cause worse GI symptoms such as cramping and loose stools. Many other "natural herbal products" have been promoted for constipation. For example, milk thistle, senna, and aloe have all been touted for their laxative properties. It is our recommendation to avoid these products. Some have been found to contain other ingredients. Even if the products are pure, they are less than ideal and they can act as stimulant laxatives, which are not nearly as safe or free of side effects as the above-mentioned nonstimulant laxatives.

What about Probiotics?

Probiotics are a concentrated form of the "good bacteria" which can normally be found in the GI tract. Different products contain diverse strains of various bacteria such as lactobacillus that may help promote GI health. These are the good bacteria commonly advertised in yogurt but found in much greater abundance in pill form. There is some research to suggest that taking these good bacteria can significantly improve GI symptoms in a variety of people: specifically those with IBD, diarrhea due to antibiotics or a viral illness, and/ or IBS. This is a very individual response, but many of our patients swear by probiotics and their role in GI health. Some people have different responses from different brands of products. Stay tuned for more research on bacteria in the GI tract. It is very possible that in the near future we will be manipulating these bacteria to help treat everything from obesity to mental illness!

Back to our patient . . . after adjusting her diet and adding magnesium, she made great progress. She's like a new woman. Sticking to this regimen, she feels better and more energized—and in turn this has motivated her to exercise more. She even lost a few pounds! Increasing the fiber in her diet eliminated her issues with hard and infrequent bowel movements, and at the same time she stopped having those occasional episodes of diarrhea. The new regimen seemed to get her GI tract "trained" so that the frequency of her bowel movements was more regulated. This is one of the great paradoxes of treating IBS—people are afraid to take something like fiber, which is known to alleviate constipation, if they are having a problem with too frequent stools. However, it is generally worth a try, because it is the bulking effect of the fiber that somehow retrains the colon to move stool through in a regular fashion. It may seem counterintuitive, but it often works!

Constipation and irritable bowel symptoms can be very unpleasant and are so common. The good news is that unlike many other more serious health issues, they are often treatable with the employment of a range of good habits and some supplements. As illustrated by our patient, a quick overhaul of one's diet and other lifestyle factors and the addition of a few off-the-shelf products can make a huge difference. So next time you feel that things are not normal with your GI tract, consider these simple and natural solutions: fiber, water, exercise, magnesium, fish oil, and probiotics.

CHAPTER 9
HORMONES GALORE
MENOPAUSE, SEX DRIVE, AND MORE

EVER HEAR SOMEONE refer to herself as "hormonal"? Ever feel like your "hormones are out of whack" or wonder if you have "hormone imbalance?" These are some of the common concerns we hear about every day. Sometimes they are grounded in real hormone-related issues that should be corrected; other times they are responses to typical bodily processes (such as aging or menopause) that can be improved upon, but not "cured."

Where to begin? Hormones are a huge part of our bodies' functioning. They are in fact so essential to our proper existence that not one but at least two entire fields of medicine have been devoted to the study of hormones (endocrinology and gynecology). Needless to say, a comprehensive review of the role of hormones in our daily lives is way beyond the scope of this book. What we do hope to do here is clarify some of the most common confusion we see in regard to endocrine-related issues, the role of vitamins and supplements in their treatment, and some pitfalls many of our patients typically run into when they read advice on the Internet or listen to some of the daytime talk shows. We would like to offer some sensible solutions to these problems that are unlikely to cause harm and more often help ease the distress of some of these issues.

Our hormones sometimes must strike a delicate balance for us to feel our best, and it is not uncommon for one of these imbalances to occur simultaneously with others. Keep this in mind as you read on. Each person's unique constellation of issues should be looked at comprehensively, and sometimes small imbalances in multiple systems can add up to big symptoms. Sometimes the best solutions are those that involve multiple incremental changes in both lifestyle and medication or over-the-counter supplements. Small changes can add up to big success if done thoughtfully and carefully.

This chapter will focus on the most common concerns related to female hormones, specifically menopause and issues related to sex drive or libido. The next chapter will focus on other endocrine issues, which involve hormonal issues that are not specific to women, such as thyroid issues and disorders of the adrenal glands.

Menopause: Is It Hot in Here, or Is It Just Me?

There's no place we'd rather start our discussion about hormones than by addressing the question, "What happens when you don't have enough of them?" The answer is menopause! Once innocuously referred to as "the change," this normal phase of life can be very dramatic. Or not. The experience varies drastically from person to person.

Menopause is, by definition, the cessation of a woman's normal monthly menstrual period. The average age of menopause is fifty. However, sometimes the perimenopausal years can run for many years before or after this magic age. Thus, we see women from ages forty to sixty dealing with some aspects of menopausal issues.

The hallmark of this natural process is the loss of the body's production of estrogen and progesterone. Once vital to a woman's fertility and monthly hormonal cycle, their production drops off significantly as the eggs in the ovaries start to peter out. This leads not only to less of these circulating hormones, but also to less testosterone, which the body had previously converted from estrogen (women of course tend to have far lower testosterone levels than men at all times). The good news is monthly bleeding comes to a halt (of course this is often after several months to years of erratic, unpredictable, and sometimes heavier periods).

The effects of losing these hormones (namely estrogen) can be profound. Hot flashes happen for many. They can range from occasional and mild to severe, frequent, and debilitating. They tend to occur more commonly at night. We hear stories of women who were cold all their lives suddenly shedding the covers at night and wrestling with their partners to turn down the thermostat. Other than the obvious benefit of saving on your heating bill, hot flashes can be highly disruptive and a source of great distress for many women.

The effects of these flushing sensations are sometimes even more wide reaching than meets the eye. They can happen at night on a more minor level, where you are not even consciously aware that they are happening. The result can be severely disrupted sleep (again this may not be obvious when it is occurring) and profound fatigue or irritability the next day. Hot flashes (whether you are aware of them or not) are often the cause for some of the common complaints associated with menopause: feeling tired, moody, and irritable; memory loss; and weight gain. The weight gain can be multifactorial, but (as we will see in our Sleep chapter) disrupted sleep does influence weight by disrupting some hormones that are key to weight and metabolism.

What to do? Menopause is a complicated issue, and, as with most issues, there is no one-size-fits-all answer. Until the late 1990s it was common practice to give women hormone replacement therapy (HRT) once they entered menopause. It made sense: replace what's missing and you can just pretend "the change" never happened. While this is so when it comes to hot flashes (they tend to disappear), there are some downsides to HRT that preclude its being an ideal solution for every woman.

HRT typically consists of replacing estrogen and progesterone at low doses with prescription doses of either hormones in either oral-, cream-, or patch-delivery systems. Estrogen is most helpful in reducing menopausal symptoms, but in women who have a uterus (i.e., those who have not had a hysterectomy) it is important that they receive progesterone with the estrogen to prevent cancer of the lining of the uterus, which can result from estrogen by itself (called "unopposed estrogen," since the progesterone controls the growth of the lining of the uterus that estrogen causes).

Estrogen and progesterone together, or combined therapy, have some pros and some cons. Relief from hot flashes and other symptoms is a big plus. Other benefits include improvement in bone density (more on this in the Bone Health chapter) and improved vaginal health (less dryness and atrophy of tissues), which can help with some aspects of urinary incontinence as well.

As with any medication, there are always potential side effects. Even this replacement of hormones the body naturally produces, when given therapeutically, turns out not to be the fountain of youth upon which many have hung their hopes. The Women's Health Initiative, a large series of studies examining these very issues, came up with some conclusions about the drawbacks of HRT. The group of women taking the estrogen and progesterone combo did end up with higher rates of heart attacks, strokes, blood clots, and breast and colon cancer. The estrogen-only group (no progesterone used because of no uterus) had increased risk of stroke and blood clot, but no change in risk of heart disease or colon cancer. The effect of estrogen only on breast cancer is still unclear, with some data suggesting a slight protective effect as compared with the harmful effect of combined therapy.

So what is the takeaway? This data suggests that hormone replacement should certainly not be used across the board in menopausal women. And while it is useful in treating bone density and hot flashes, the increased risk of cardiovascular problems and malignancies suggests very judicious use is prudent. It is our practice to recommend HRT only to women who have intolerable menopausal symptoms that are not amenable to other therapies (more on what those might be later). They should use the lowest dose possible and for the least amount of time possible. The use of topical estrogens for vaginal dryness is of less concern since they are considered to act locally and not be systemically absorbed.

A very popular practice since the mid-2000s has been the use of "bioidentical hormones," which are compounded hormones given in varying doses on an individual basis, either in the form of pills, patches, or gels. This practice often includes the use of estrogen, progesterone, testosterone, and DHEA in varying amounts.

In theory, we love the idea that we are not all the same and each have different individual needs. In fact, one of our founding missions at Vous Vitamin® has been to address people's individual needs in regard to vitamins. However, we do not believe the science currently supports these particular methods of hormone replacement.

There are no significant studies that show any benefit to these over traditional hormones; and especially given the varied methods, absorption, and general lack of standardization in these practices, it is very hard to safely recommend them. The use of testosterone and DHEA are actually not FDA approved for use in women at all. Also, there is no standardization to the methods by which individuals are measured and applied to therapy. In fact, studies have shown that there is little correlation between hormone levels and actual menopausal symptoms. Using these levels to target therapies, then, does not make logical sense. Therefore, we advise extreme caution in the use of "bioidenticals." We understand that many women swear by the wonderful effects on their hot flashes, sex drive, and more. However, we believe many of these issues can be remedied with more proven, potentially safer means, both prescription and not.

So what to do about menopausal symptoms? There are some prescription and natural remedies with decent evidence in their favor. First, we need to recognize that menopausal symptoms naturally resolve on their own in the vast majority of people. Most women's symptoms abate within two to five years of onset. However, a small percentage, less than 10 percent, will continue to have hot flashes ten years into menopause and beyond.

If the symptoms are troublesome, some prescription options (other than hormones) can be considered, namely a variety of antidepressants. The key here is to recognize that they can be used in menopause beyond their use for depression. Some of the SSRIs and SNRIs (common classes of antianxiety/antidepressants) are very helpful in reducing hot flashes. We prefer SNRIs, as they tend to have fewer side effects (weight gain and loss of libido are more common with SSRIs). Venlafaxine and the other drugs in this class can be helpful in reducing hot flashes and some of the mood symptoms often associated with menopause.

Some herbal remedies are also commonly used for hot flashes. Perhaps the most popular is black cohosh. This root, from a plant native to North America, is touted as a natural reducer of hot flashes and vaginal dryness. While studies are mixed as to whether or not it is helpful, we have found that in practice it is hit or miss. That is, some women find it very helpful in reducing symptoms while others do not. As for any downsides, it is generally considered safe. However, rare reports of liver problems have been made. It is our belief that finding a pure reputable brand is essential as with all herbal and supplement products. Some authorities also caution using black cohosh if you have a history of breast cancer due to concerns that it may stimulate estrogen receptors. Data on this is lacking, but we do advise finding another solution in women with a family history of breast cancer.

Vitamin E has been indicated as playing a role in reducing hot flashes. Some studies have combined it with black cohosh to show some modest relief, even at lower doses. It is our belief that low doses of vitamin E (under 100 IUs) are generally safe and possibly useful. Higher doses can increase risk of bleeding and have not been shown to be more effective.

Phytoestrogens (plant-derived xenoestrogens) have been shown to reduce some symptoms of menopause. Since many can be found in natural food sources (soy products abound), we suggest obtaining soy in moderation through these products (not to exceed two servings daily) and avoiding supplementation. Because soy and phytoestrogens can have an effect on estrogen receptors, caution should be used especially among those with a breast cancer history.

Both primrose oil and flaxseed have been suggested for hot flashes. Little evidence supports their use. We believe you can do better with some of the other treatments mentioned.

Last but certainly not least talked about is DHEA. Many tout this supplement for its role in stopping aging or improving sex drive. If you think it sounds too good to be true, you are probably right.

DHEA is a hormone made by the body in the adrenal gland, a small gland that rests on top of the kidney. It's a building block used by your body to make other sex hormones like testosterone and estrogen. DHEA gradually declines with age after peaking in your twenties. While DHEA supplementation has been shown to improve bone density, its effect on hot flashes and other libido issues has not been proven. What does seem likely is an association between high DHEA levels and breast cancer. It is also known to cause hair loss. Therefore, we do not find its use warranted. Too bad; so sad: DHEA is not the fountain of youth. It sounds way better than it actually performs.

Menopause is a natural phase of life but is nonetheless a disruption of a woman's previous hormonal balance that can cause many negative symptoms. However, most women can weather the storm and find a new and pleasant normal once hot flashes subside. There are many prescription and vitamin or supplement options for helping women through this period of flux. Hormone replacement is a complicated consideration, and each woman's risks and benefits should be assessed individually. While menopause is a universal process, each woman's experience with it is unique and should be treated as such.

The Low Libido

A common complaint among both women and men is low sex drive. We often hear this from women, starting in their thirties and progressing with age, who feel their libido is in decline. The cause is usually related to several factors, some psychological and some physical or hormone related.

Firstly, let us be clear that any disruption in the normal cycling and ebb and flow of hormones can affect sex drive. If you think about it from both a psychological and an evolutionary standpoint, our bodies only want to reproduce when conditions are ideal (at least most women we talk to feel that way). Men tend to be a bit less particular about the circumstances.

This means that, for example, when your thyroid is not functioning properly, or you are perimenopausal or experiencing menopause, the fluctuation in these other hormones can affect the hormones that drive libido. The female body doesn't find itself in the mood too often when it's experiencing hot flashes, premenstrual syndrome (PMS), or other hormone-driven unpleasantness.

So, the first step in examining low libido is to investigate other hormonal issues. These can be normal processes such as PMS or menopause, or pathological problems such as a low or overactive thyroid or more rare pituitary issues (which should be looked into by a physician). One nice gauge for whether or not things in your endocrine system are functioning smoothly in younger women is the monthly menstrual cycle. If you are reliably getting a monthly period, it is less likely (though not impossible) that you have a major problem with your endocrine system. Your body reserves fertility for times when everything is functioning well. So the presence of a monthly period, which typically means you are ovulating (unless you are on birth control pills), is one sign that things are working as they should be.

If hormones are generally in balance, sex drive may be diminished for other reasons. Fatigue is a common one. New mothers often experience this. They sometimes lose interest in sex for many months to years after having a baby. Their partners are perplexed. We see and hear this all the time from our patients. Most of the time the cause is simple: fatigue. These women are exhausted from having a newborn then a toddler. They are chronically sleep deprived, stressed out, and malnourished (more on this soon). They are essentially in survival mode; it is no wonder that sexual interludes are not their first priority during those precious uninterrupted moments in bed. Generally sleep is.

Women in perimenopause are sometimes in a similar situation. They may be experiencing hot flashes, which disrupt their sleep (whether they are aware or not) and lead to fatigue and irritability.

This moves sexual interest down on their list somewhat. Once women enter menopause, their interest can take a serious decline for these reasons as well as a drop in estrogen and testosterone. Testosterone is the hormonal trigger for sex drive, so its decline naturally can reduce libido. The lack of estrogen can take its toll by causing vaginal dryness and atrophy, which tends to make the act less comfortable even if the drive is there.

Sounding pretty hopeless? Fear not. A few interventions, some medical and some involving vitamins, can be of use. Of course, correcting any true endocrine issue (like thyroid problems) should take precedence. Once that has been done, addressing any menopausal issues is also important. As previously discussed, hormone replacement is a mixed bag and it is not without potential downsides. For some women, it can be tremendously helpful in this arena. For others, not as much. Each individual must decide with their physician's help if it is the right choice for them. Testosterone cream is commonplace these days for this indication, though the FDA has not approved its use in women.

One supplement often touted as useful for libido is DHEA. (See our previous discussion above, in the menopause section.) There is inconclusive evidence to support the role of DHEA in treating low libido. There is also a significant association between higher levels of DHEA and breast cancer. For these reasons we do not recommend its use.

There are some supplements and vitamins that can be useful for sex drive. For centuries, Asian cultures have used ginseng to enhance libidinal drive in men and women. There is some good research in both animals and people that it can increase sex drive and sexual activity.

Some sources also recommend low doses of caffeine. This may simply work to combat the snooze effect. In other words, if you are more alert and awake, you may resist the urge to collapse into sleep and in turn this may translate into putting you in the mood. On that note, any of the strategies discussed in the Energy and Fatigue chapter (specifically iron, B vitamins, and vitamin D) can come into play. Feeling your best all around can go a long way in the bedroom.

Hormonal issues of all kinds can really rock your world if things are not properly balanced. Menopause leaves its calling card for most women in the form of hot flashes and more. It's rare to get through "the change" without some notable symptoms, though there is a huge range as to how much it takes its toll on daily life. Likewise, libido issues can be a huge problem for some and less so for others. We think that both issues are best dealt with through education about why you are experiencing symptoms and knowing more about available prescription, over-the-counter, and lifestyle options for treating them. Vitamins and supplements can be a piece of the equation and a part of the solution that helps many women feel like themselves again.

CHAPTER 10
ENDOCRINOLOGY AND METABOLISM 101

COMMON MISCONCEPTIONS ABOUT GLANDULAR PROBLEMS

WE WOULD BE COMPLETELY off base to suggest that most endocrine disorders can be treated with vitamins. However, what we have found is that many issues commonly misconstrued as endocrine problems are in fact vitamin deficiencies masquerading as these other diagnoses. We would like to help dispel some of the most common misunderstandings we see in our practices.

An in-depth education on endocrinology is clearly beyond the reach of this book. Romy, in fact, spent an extra two years in training focusing on issues related to glands and the hormones they produce. Clearly, there are many nuances to understanding this body system, but for the purposes of this chapter we would like to focus on a few misconceptions we see repeatedly among our patients and some of the ways we think their symptoms can be better addressed. Namely, we will delve into concerns about the thyroid and adrenal glands.

Our Theory of the Thyroid

Perhaps one of the most common disorders that our patients self-diagnose is a low thyroid. It seems that just about everyone who walks into our offices is convinced his or her thyroid is not functioning properly.

People Google search a litany of terms from "fatigue" to "trouble losing weight" to "thinning hair" and thyroid always comes up at the top of the list of potential causes.

No doubt it is an incredibly important gland, and its function is essential to your body's overall health. Romy is in fact a thyroidologist (a subspeciality within endocrinology and metabolism), and she has made a career of studying and treating this gland found in each of our necks overlying our Adam's apple (the piece of cartilage in your neck that protects your windpipe—it is more prominent in men, but every woman has one, too). Our discussion of endocrine issues and hormones certainly must shed some light on this essential and much-publicized gland. There are in fact some vitamins and supplements that are important for thyroid health and others that we believe should not be used, though are commonly recommended.

In many ways, our thyroid serves as the epicenter of metabolism in our bodies. The thyroid uses iodine (found in our diets or via supplements, more on this later) to produce a hormone, in the form of thyroxine (T4). T4 circulates and is converted throughout the body into its more active form, triiodothyronine (T3), which is the hormone responsible for essentially "keeping things going" in our bodies.

If we lack thyroid hormone (i.e., are hypothyroid), our heart rate can slow, we can gain weight, feel depressed or fatigued or cold all the time, even lose cognitive function and memory, become constipated, have erratic menstrual periods, and lose hair. Sounds great, right? However, the opposite end of the spectrum isn't so terrific either. Those who have excess thyroid hormone (i.e., are hyperthyroid) feel jumpy, get palpitations, lose bone density, feel hot all the time, and have tremors, trouble sleeping, diarrhea, and erratic periods, as well as hair loss. Clearly, living in the middle, in perfect balance, is where we all want to be.

How do we assess our thyroid status? A simple blood test will do the trick. It is our practice to screen all patients over thirty annually for thyroid disorders. Some younger patients should have occasional screening as well, especially if there is a family history of thyroid disease as it tends to run in families. There is an association between thyroid disorders and other autoimmune conditions, such as IBD, type 1 diabetes, and rheumatoid arthritis, among others.

The most useful blood test for looking at thyroid function is the thyroid-stimulating hormone (or TSH) test. It determines the blood level of the TSH hormone that the brain sends out to regulate the thyroid. If the brain senses too little circulating hormone, the TSH goes up. If it senses too much, this number goes down. For this reason, deciding if someone's thyroid is over- or underactive is a bit counter-intuitive—a low TSH means the thyroid is overactive (hyperthyroid), while a high TSH means it is underactive (hypothyroid). An under-active thyroid is by far the more common finding. Other levels, such as T4 and T3, can be used in conjunction with the TSH. Conditions typically causing under- and overactive thyroids are Hashimoto's thyroiditis and Graves' disease, respectively. These are both auto-immune conditions, which involve various antibodies attacking the thyroid gland.

If your thyroid is in fact underactive, it is generally simple to treat. We typically use synthetic thyroid (such as levothyroxine), which is a close approximate to the T4 your body makes. It is essential when taking levothyroxine to take it in the prescribed way, since it must be absorbed properly and uniformly each day; otherwise regulating thyroid levels will be difficult. T4 replacement can actually be taken any time of day as long as you are consistent about the time and way in which you take it. Thyroid hormone should be taken on an empty stomach, and you should wait thirty minutes before eating. You should also not take any vitamins (particularly those that contain iron or calcium) within three hours of taking the thyroid hormone, as they can interfere with its absorption. Same for antacids and choles-terol-lowering medications. These vitamins and medications should be avoided for three hours before and after taking the medication. Finding the right time to take your levothyroxine can be a challenge, but taking it consistently as part of a regular routine is important to get consistent absorption and blood levels.

Thyroid levels can be reassessed five to six weeks after starting thyroid replacement or changing a dose. It takes this long to see an accurate rise or fall in TSH. Remember, this is the brain's response to how much hormone it senses. Your brain takes a while to figure things out. For this reason, changes in thyroid hormone can only be assessed and adjusted after five to six weeks of treatment. This also speaks to the slow-acting nature of levothyroxine. It is metabolized slowly and has a long half-life. Therefore, its effects are felt not in minutes or hours but rather in days or weeks. You must be patient to feel its effects, but it is certainly worth it to restore your metabolism to its natural state.

We know that the Internet is ripe with tales of people's use of and the wonders of "natural thyroid products." Many tout the importance of using T3 products rather than T4. They theorize that some people cannot convert T4 to T3. Medical research tells us differently. Most people do in fact convert T4 to T3 when the T4 is replaced. It may take time to see this effect, months in fact. T3 replacement is all the rage, but not with those who actually know the research and the science concerning the thyroid. People who are truly knowledgeable of thyroid replacement, such as the American Thyroid Association, do not condone its widespread use—and for good reason. Sometimes something that sounds too good to be true is in fact too good to be true.

Replacing T3 is often done with various glandular products. These are preparations touted as a more "natural" way to replace thyroid hormones. Let us be clear here: They are not. They are in no way more physiological or natural. They are made from ground-up pig or sheep thyroid. If this itself is not unappealing enough for you, recognize that their concentration varies greatly from batch to batch because of the way glandular products are manufactured. Therefore, using these products leads to erratic regulation of the thyroid from batch to batch—i.e., one month you are taking too much, the next month not enough. Because of the lag in TSH to assess dosing success, you are constantly chasing your tail trying to find the correct dose. In addition, T3 (unlike synthetic T4) is very short acting. This means you take the pill and actually feel the effects within hours—typically a rush of energy and sometimes palpitations. However, this passes quickly and you then experience a big crash in energy. It is a roller coaster ride of sorts, with big highs and lows. There is in fact nothing natural about it, and all the perils of being both hyper- and hypothyroid can be experienced in the same day: fatigue, palpitations, tremors, and more. Synthetic T4 taken properly and monitored so that TSH is kept at a normal level is completely natural and physiologically sound, because it is exactly how your body would do it if it could. The vast majority of our patients are successfully treated with T4 replacement if properly dosed and monitored. (On rare occasions, a combination of prescription T4 and very small amounts of prescription T3 can be used.) The American Thyroid Association and Endocrine Society do not endorse the use of "glandular" products, and we decidedly agree. In our practices, we have seen numerous people over the years who have been given these products by other doctors with hopes of weight loss, energy, and other false promises. They take their T3 and get a brief rush of energy followed by a crash. Ultimately, we end up seeing them when they are exhausted and depressed. We have also seen people with serious heart complications related to the use of T3.

One vitamin that is essential to proper thyroid function is iodine (also touched on in our Energy and Fatigue chapter). Iodine is the building block the thyroid uses to produce hormones. It is common sense that we need it to keep our thyroid running properly. For the last hundred years or so this was generally not a problem in the typical American diet because with the industrialization of our food industry, table salt has been fortified with iodine. However, as many of us have strived for better health in recent years, we have largely cut table salt and processed foods out of our diets. This is generally a good thing. As we have opted for small amounts of kosher or sea salt instead of the more potent table salt, we have virtually eliminated our main source of iodine. While some other foods contain it, such as seaweed, some fish, and cranberries, many of us who do eat healthfully need an iodine supplement.

Worldwide iodine deficiency is a huge problem; and from this we know that it causes goiters (an enlargement of the thyroid), hypothyroidism, and major issues in babies and children born to mothers in an iodine-deficient state (including developmental delay and slowed growth). Therefore, it is essential that we all get enough of this vitamin. However, as with many things, too much can cause its own host of problems. Some commercially available iodine supplements sold in the name of "thyroid support" contain many hundreds of times the recommended dose. This can backfire in a big way. Too much iodine can cause inflammation of the gland and a rapid release of hormone that is both unpleasant and harmful. Needless to say, taking a safe amount of iodine is essential. We are comfortable with the recommendation of between 150 and 220 mcg of supplemental iodine daily (the higher end of this range is needed by pregnant and nursing women). We have been careful at Vous Vitamin® to include it in safe doses in our multivitamin formulations.

Another supplement that is often found in discussions of thyroid health is L-carnitine. It turns out this amino acid has some effect in blocking the effects of T3 and T4. It is therefore recommended for those with Graves' disease (the most typical cause of an overactive thyroid). However, its effect is limited at best, and if anything L-carnitine could be useful as an adjunct to legitimate medical treatment for this condition (the specifics of this are beyond the scope of this book, but suffice it to say, hyperthyroidism should be treated by a medical doctor with FDA-approved therapies).

There is some buzz about the mineral selenium, and it playing a role in autoimmune thyroid conditions. Though it has been suggested to help with both hypo- and hyperthyroidism, as of 2014 there is no conclusive evidence to suggest it can be routinely and safely used for thyroid disease. Its biggest role may be in treating some of the effects of Graves' disease on the eyes. Taking selenium should be done under the guidance of a physician.

The thyroid is an important and much talked about gland. The good news is that supporting it with the proper amount of iodine is fairly simple (just beware of too much). When abnormalities occur that are not due to iodine deficiency, such as hypo- or hyperthyroidism, treatment with FDA-approved therapies is advised. We strongly discourage the "glandular" preparations, despite their being touted as a more "natural" approach. Their effect on metabolism is in fact anything but natural.

The Truth about Your Adrenal Glands and Fatigue

The term "adrenal fatigue" is all the rage these days. Everyone from holistic doctors to massage therapists to yoga instructors seems to throw it around like crazy. According to many, it explains why people feel poorly and can be simply remedied with a dose of either DHEA and/or certain "physiological steroids." We beg to differ.

We by no means wish to cast judgment on the above-mentioned practitioners. We are simply noting that this diagnosis seems to be made by a litany of people, yet by very few (if any) legitimately trained, board-certified endocrinologists (doctors of medicine who specialize in glands and hormones, including the adrenal gland). Perhaps this is because it is not actually a medically sound diagnosis.

Adrenal fatigue is, however, based on some legitimate medical concepts, and it is perhaps loosely related to the very real condition of adrenal insufficiency. We will first explain what the adrenal gland is and does, then delve into these malfunctions of it. We will also explain how the phenomenon of "adrenal fatigue" may be explained by some vitamin deficiencies and other conditions, and how to treat it accordingly.

The adrenal glands are small organs that sit on top of your kidneys. They pack a big punch for glands the size of your thumbs. The adrenals produce many hormones that are vital to our bodies functioning properly. Specifically they produce steroid hormones and adrenaline-type hormones. DHEA (mentioned previously in reference to libido) is one of the steroid-hormone precursors (building blocks).

The steroid hormones consist of aldosterone, testosterone, and cortisol. Aldosterone and testosterone regulate blood pressure and sex drive. Cortisol is considered a "stress hormone." This very important hormone is secreted by your adrenals during times of stress and, accordingly, it helps sustain various parts of your metabolism at those times—i.e., it helps keep blood pressure and blood sugar up (since they are likely to drop if you are starving or bleeding). Cortisol is in fact the reason why most people do not actually get drops in blood sugar when they are hungry (even if they experience the symptoms associated with low sugar). Our naturally produced steroid hormones are some of our best defenses against illness and injury.

The adrenaline hormones are also used in times of stress. Remember that whole fight-or-flight thing from science class? These are the hormones that make your heart beat faster when a bear is about to attack you. These hormones also go crazy when you are riled up.

Clearly if the adrenals are out of whack one way or the other, you've got problems. If your adrenals are overactive (typically caused by a tumor of some kind) and you get lots of these stress-type hormones circulating, predictably, you get the symptoms of feeling stressed—fast heart rate, high blood pressure, sometimes a flushing reaction—even when you shouldn't be. In the case of cortisol, you can experience sugars that are too high, weight gain, hair loss, and even anxiety and/or depression. This can be called either Cushing's syndrome or pheochromocytoma, depending on which part of the gland is overproducing (complicated stuff that's kind of beyond our scope here). Needless to say, this is not an enjoyable state of affairs; and these are serious, but exceedingly rare, conditions.

If your adrenals are underactive, you have different issues. In the medical community this is referred to as adrenal insufficiency, and it typically occurs due to an autoimmune condition where your body actually makes antibodies against your adrenal glands or due to long-term use of oral steroids (like prednisone) for other conditions, which essentially stops your glands from working on their own. There are other very rare causes such as bleeding into the glands or tumors that replace the glands. All of these are very unusual but potentially life-threatening conditions, because, as we explained previously, your body relies on these glands during times of stress. And stress is a relative term; it can even refer to having a cold or a low-grade fever. If the adrenals are not making aldosterone and cortisol, your blood pressure can drop as a result and you can pass out, or even worse.

This is a medical emergency. People who have true (or suspected) adrenal insufficiency need medical evaluation and treatment. These patients respond dramatically (within minutes to hours to adrenal replacement—they nearly rise from the dead with a dose of steroids). The protocols for treatment typically consist of intravenous steroids in the emergent situation followed by lifelong oral steroids (such as prednisone). People with adrenal insufficiency should also wear medical alert bracelets so that in case of an emergency, providers know to dose them with IV steroids. This can be very scary stuff to be sure.

What we have just described is adrenal insufficiency. In contrast, the lay media makes common reference to the term adrenal fatigue. The theory behind adrenal fatigue is that if we have lots of stress we "use up" all of the stress hormones that our adrenals make and they somehow wear out. Sounds plausible, but yet it does not bear out scientifically. This term has been used to explain a whole host of symptoms from fatigue to irritability to GI symptoms, body aches, and more. It is unclear to us how it is diagnosed since there are no gold standard or data-proven tests (true adrenal insufficiency is diagnosed with what's called a stimulation test). Various online questionnaires to see if you have adrenal fatigue tend to ask about amounts of stress and fatigue that one experiences. Some practitioners tout saliva, blood, and urine testing, but they do not use the medically proven diagnostic test that includes giving a dose of hormone to stimulate the adrenals and then testing their response.

With a vague definition and unclear means of diagnosing this entity, it is not surprising that there are a wide variety of recommendations for treating adrenal fatigue. A huge selection of supplements is pedaled for its use, including everything from standard vitamins to heavy metals and glandular preparations (again, concoctions made from ground-up animal glands). Some include DHEA. Some do not.

The real medical data suggest something different. If you are in a constant state of stress, your adrenals actually gear up and *overproduce* stress hormones such as cortisol. Your glands make too much of these hormones and you get all of the unfortunate side effects of too much steroid—thin hair, weight gain, trouble sleeping, feeling exhausted (because the "rush of energy" can go only so far, you do ultimately crash). Therefore, why would one try to treat this overstressed condition with even more stress hormones? Even worse, the long-term use of steroids includes the side effect of shutting down your own body's normal production of cortisol, which can be dangerous. When this happens, the body cannot naturally raise its cortisol response during illness or emergencies, and disaster can ensue.

The concept of adrenal fatigue is so appealing. It seems to be something we could all say we have. We are tired; we are stressed; we have moments of feeling poorly. So many of us have various symptoms that are not easily explained, and it is somehow reassuring to think that there is a quick fix for this. Certainly, there are solutions to symptoms caused by stress and fatigue. There is no doubt that "burning the candle at both ends" takes its toll on our bodies, and this must be addressed.

However, the bottom line is that we are tired of adrenal fatigue. When there is no objective way to diagnose or treat a condition, it's hard to accept it as valid. This was nicely stated by Mayo Clinic endocrinologist Dr. Todd B. Nippoldt: "It's frustrating to have persistent symptoms your doctor can't readily explain. But accepting a medically unrecognized diagnosis from an unqualified practitioner could be worse."

We are highly skeptical of this diagnosis. Rather, we believe the symptoms that may lead one to consider it are very real and certainly should be explored. Of the many patients over the years who have come to us on various regimens for adrenal fatigue, most have been on a host of glandular preparations. A few have been on actual prednisone or other prescription steroids, rarely with any legitimate testing to justify their use. Many have had side effects from the "treatment" they were taking, which they attributed to their underlying condition—weight gain, hair loss, anxiety, a rush of energy followed by profound fatigue, high blood sugars, and more. Sometimes it is hard to even know with what problem they actually started.

After ruling out other medical conditions it has been our experience that many of these people suffer from classic vitamin deficiencies, typically those that cause fatigue and lack of energy (see the chapter dedicated to this subject). It can take months to see the effects of the other treatments wearing off and to adequately replete iron, vitamin D, various B vitamins, and magnesium. Eventually most people end up feeling much better once they have simplified their vitamin regimen and gotten back to a healthy routine—adequate sleep, a good diet, and a regular exercise regimen.

It is true that stress causes cortisol levels to rise. This is not good for you for many, many reasons: It contributes to obesity, poor sleep, etc. However, 99 percent of us have fully functional adrenal glands despite major stressors. Those of us whose adrenals fail do not have this problem because of stress and do need a legitimate endocrine evaluation by a certified endocrinologist.

The rest of us need to take a step back and first of all try to troubleshoot the sources of our anxiety. We cannot always change external circumstances, but we can do our part to change how we process them. We can teach ourselves techniques such as mindfulness and meditation, and even consider individual therapy to work through some of our issues and decompress by sharing our perspective with an objective outsider (rather than a friend or family member). We can take care of ourselves in addition to others by allowing ourselves the time to sleep, exercise, and eat properly. These are the backbone of a healthy and lower-stress existence. We can also replenish our nutritional needs with proper vitamin supplementation based on our individual requirements (see more in our Energy and Fatigue chapter as well as the Vitamin Glossary).

Taking ground-up adrenal glands from an animal is no way to address your own symptoms associated with stress and exhaustion. Your symptoms should be examined carefully and treated with thought and care by an experienced practitioner in combination with the above-mentioned lifestyle changes as well as a safe and thoughtful vitamin regimen.

———————◦♦◦———————

We have given you an overview of some of the most common endocrine-related concerns that we encounter in practice. Clearly, how our glands regulate our body's normal balance is a complicated business that plays a huge role in how we feel and how we function every day. Subtle changes can sometimes have big effects. It is important, though, not to attribute every unusual feeling or symptom to a glandular problem. Issues related to endocrine imbalances are typically quantifiably diagnosed and treated by a physician.

There is a role for vitamins and supplements in addressing some of the deficiencies that often cause these symptoms and in supporting your glands to function at their best. However, it is important to be educated and safe when using over-the-counter products for these purposes, as sometimes taking the wrong products can be unsafe and potentially worsen the situation. Glandular replacement products are often fraught with inconsistencies in manufacturing and potentially dangerous side effects, and they should be avoided.

Thyroid disorders and adrenal issues are very real matters that plague many people. However, if they are ruled out by a reliable practitioner, other causes for symptoms should be entertained. Vitamins and supplements should be used to replace common deficiencies in nutrients that we need. These measures, in addition to changes to sleep habits, stress reduction, exercise, and diet, can also play an essential role in feeling better.

CHAPTER 11

VITAMINS FOR IMMUNITY AND BODY ACHES

CURING WHAT AILS YOU

INVARIABLY WE ALL HAVE DAYS when we feel like we are falling apart. These seem to increase as we get older; but even at young ages, many of us have aches and pains, sniffles and sore throats, or other unpleasant symptoms that can really put a damper on our activities. When we lead active lives, we are prone to injury; or sometimes things happen spontaneously. Likewise, common respiratory illnesses often occur through one's exposure to lots of people or seem to materialize from nowhere. Either way, vitamins play a part in handling these common complaints.

In this chapter, we will delve into immunity first and discuss how we can all improve our health to minimize infections. Later on, we will move on to body aches and vitamins' key role in preventing and easing these symptoms. Certain vitamins and supplements can be an essential part of lifestyle changes that help you feel your best more often.

There are times when it can feel like everyone is coughing and sneezing all around you. When cold season gets into full swing, we all look for ways not to get sick. As physicians and mothers of young children, we are on the frontlines of illness and feel like we are showered with germs each day. The new millennium has brought epidemics, including swine flu (H1N1), influenza, enterovirus,

whooping cough, measles, Ebola, and more. It's easy to get para-
noid about catching something, but we can't live in a bubble.
We can, however, all take some simple measures to avoid getting
unnecessarily ill, including making a number of lifestyle changes
and learning about what vitamins can play an important role in
building your defenses against disease.

Simple hand washing is probably the easiest thing we can do.
Avoid touching surfaces such as doorknobs and then touching your
face. Also wash your hands regularly before eating. Antibacterial gels
can be used. However, the old-fashioned method of washing hands
with warm water and soap is the preferred method to avoid alcohol
and other harsh chemicals in these gels. Using the trick of singing
"Happy Birthday" while washing ensures you devote adequate time to
the task. Likewise, prevent the spread of your own germs by coughing
or sneezing into your elbow rather than your hands.

Another habit that can help boost our immunity is getting a
good amount of sleep. You've heard us harp on sleep before, but it
is so important to allow your body that restorative time. Sleep is a
useful way for your body to refuel and build up all of its best defenses
against illness. Sleep deprivation may play a role in lowering one's
immune strength. It certainly contributes to other conditions such as
obesity and diabetes, which are associated with higher rates of certain
infections.

Stress reduction may also be important in protecting our immune
system. Numerous studies have shown that higher levels of stress lead
to more frequent and worse infections. This is likely due to production
of cortisol, the body's main stress hormone. In the short term, cortisol
helps us power through stress; but in the long term, ongoing high
levels of cortisol tend to open us up to infections.

Other lifestyle measures that are known to help reduce rates
of infection are stopping smoking and minimizing alcohol intake.
Smoking impairs the lungs, sinuses, and upper airways in their ability
to rid themselves of harmful bacteria; therefore quitting (at any stage
in life) is worthwhile. Likewise, alcohol impairs the body's natural
abilities to fight infection. Chronic alcohol consumption diminishes

the white blood cells' functions and decreases the immune system's strength. Too bad the old wives' tale about a "hot brandy" to cure what ails you has been put to rest!

No responsible discussion of fighting infection would be complete without mention of age-appropriate vaccination. Vaccination is perhaps the most proven way to reduce the rates and severity of infection from a variety of illnesses, including influenza, whooping cough, measles, pneumococcal pneumonia, and more. Discuss appropriate vaccination practices with your health-care provider.

When it comes to vitamins for immune health, the most commonly talked about vitamin for preventing colds is vitamin C. This water-soluble vitamin is found in citrus fruits, berries, tomatoes, broccoli, bell peppers, and many other fruits and vegetables. While its exact role in immunity has been long debated, vitamin C's antioxidant properties may help with healing and disease fighting. We know it is helpful in skin, wound, and bone healing for these reasons. There is research to suggest that vitamin C does help shorten the duration of colds; and some studies suggest it can help prevent colds, especially among those who are in cold environments or who exercise strenuously. There does not appear to be a great benefit to using supplemental doses higher than 500 mg daily. And there are potential side effects from using too much, such as GI symptoms and kidney stones. For these reasons, we believe it is reasonable to supplement with a daily dose of approximately 250 mg and perhaps step it up to 500 mg daily with the onset of respiratory or other infectious symptoms. While many popular over-the-counter immune supplements boast blends of vitamins including C for immunity, our experience with them is that they tend to contain too much of certain vitamins and not enough of others. They often are high in vitamin A, which can be potentially harmful (see Vitamin Glossary for details).

Another vitamin that seems to improve immunity is vitamin D3. One of our favorites, this fat-soluble vitamin seems to play a role in disease prevention in that its deficiency is associated with higher rates of illness. Even centuries ago people treated tuberculosis with sunlight (this likely worked because sunlight stimulates vitamin D production in the body). While conclusive studies have not been conducted to link using supplements to preventing the common cold, it makes intuitive sense that this important vitamin should be taken to prevent deficiency. Unfortunately, most of us are deficient in this vitamin. Vitamin D's main source is the sun, and the majority of us live in climates that do not provide adequate year-round sun exposure and/ or we wisely use sun protection to avoid other damaging effects, such as skin cancer and wrinkles. A few foods naturally contain vitamin D (wild-caught salmon and calf liver), but these do not tend to be staples in our diets. Milk and orange juice are fortified with it, but usually not in significant quantities. Therefore, we believe that vitamin D (as its most active form, D3) should be a part of most people's vitamin regimens. Exact amounts to take can range depending on where you live, your diet, and other health concerns (such as conditions like celiac disease that impair absorption).

Zinc's role in decreasing the duration of the common cold has been explored and validated. Zinc is an elemental metal that appears to have some effect on reducing the rhinovirus (a common virus that causes colds). We know it can also be helpful in wound healing, so there may be a role for zinc in helping tissues to return to normal. We are not advocates of daily zinc for cold prevention since over-supplementation with heavy metals may be toxic. Rather, we think it is most useful as an occasional as-needed supplement when we are most at risk for an illness. For example, taking zinc may be helpful for several days after being exposed to an illness or at the onset of an infection. At Vous Vitamin®, we created our Immune Blast™ supplement based on this principle. It is a blend of zinc, vitamin D, and vitamin C that is intended for use with exposure to illness or at the onset respiratory symptoms. It comes in a pocket-size packet to keep on hand for when needed.

A variety of herbs have been suggested to play a role in immunity, namely aloe vera, echinacea, and ginseng. Unfortunately, the data is not compelling enough for us to recommend their routine use for this purpose. They are likely not harmful if you find a pure source from a reputable manufacturer, but we do not believe they are worth the effort or expense. Probiotics can certainly be helpful for recovering from GI illnesses and prevention of certain bacterial infections of the gut. (See our chapter on Constipation and IBS for more on this topic.)

All in all, there are certainly measures one can take to minimize the risk of getting or staying sick. Common sense strategies such as hand washing, vaccination, and getting enough sleep are sure to help fortify your body's ability to fight disease. Certain vitamins can also be helpful when used properly.

Body Aches

We frequently see people in our practice who come in complaining, "I am turning forty, but I feel like I'm ninety. My whole body hurts all the time. If I injure myself exercising, it takes so long to get better." Aches and pains are to some extent a normal part of aging, but steps should be taken to address and minimize them whenever possible. While medical conditions can be a cause for pain and should be ruled out, vitamins can often play a role in helping to alleviate these symptoms.

The first consideration is whether your discomfort is in your joints or your muscles. Aching joints can be caused by a host of medical conditions (including osteoarthritis, the typical wear-and-tear arthritis), as well as a number of inflammatory arthritis conditions (including but not limited to rheumatoid arthritis and lupus). These should be investigated by your doctor. Vitamins may play a useful adjunctive role in treating painful joints.

Body aches can also be muscular in origin. It is worth exploring causes for muscle aches with your doctor as they too can be caused by treatable conditions such as thyroid disorders, autoimmune conditions, and more. Musculoskeletal aches also can be attributed to deficiencies in certain important vitamins and electrolytes.

We will first discuss arthritis and the many supplements that have been recommended to treat it. Arthritis is a condition caused by the breakdown of cartilage. Cartilage is the smooth squishy substance that cushions your joints at the intersection of two bones. The resulting breakdown of cartilage causes pain, typically with movement of the joint. There is often swelling as well. Arthritis may sound like an ailment specific to the elderly, but it is in fact a condition that can start as early as thirty in some people. The list of supplements that have been suggested for this very common condition is exhaustive; however, the number of supplements with good evidence and good safety profiles is more limited. As with most vitamin choices, each person has unique needs and responds differently to different things.

Some of the most commonly talked-about supplements are glucosamine and chondroitin. Glucosamine is an amino sugar found in joint fluid. It is one of the building blocks of cartilage. Chondroitin is a sugar compound that is an important component of cartilage and other connective tissues. Each of these compounds can be given as supplements with the intention of treating arthritic pain. In theory, they help rebuild damaged cartilage. Data suggests that the two taken together (less so taken individually) can be useful in reducing the symptoms of arthritic pain. Our experience with patients taking these products tells us that they can be very helpful in reducing some people's symptoms. However, this is not a uniform experience for all people, and some do not find glucosamine and/or chondroitin that helpful. The downsides are minimal since side effects are rarely reported.

Another supplement that has been touted for this issue is SAMe (short for S-adenosylmethionine). There are some studies suggesting it can be as effective as some anti-inflammatory medications. However, caution should be used with this supplement since it can cause both GI side effects as well as have significant interactions with antidepressant medications.

Vitamin C is an antioxidant, and it is known to play an important role in building connective tissue, including the collagen found in cartilage. In theory it should help with arthritic complaints. It has in fact been shown that people with less vitamin C in their diet are more likely to develop arthritis. However, the data for using vitamin C as treatment is lacking. That being said, it is our opinion that supplementing with low-dose vitamin C is worth a try for those who suffer from arthritic pain. A generally acceptable dose that is unlikely to cause harm is 250–500 mg daily.

Known for their role in fighting inflammation are the omega-3s found in either fish oil or flaxseed oil. These supplements are thus likely to be more useful in fighting arthritis caused by inflammatory conditions. Another big player in the anti-inflammatory world is turmeric. Turmeric, or curcumin, has long been used in Chinese and Indian ayurvedic medicine. Around 2010 it became more popular in traditional circles due to some good data suggesting it can help with arthritis symptoms. Turmeric can be found naturally (as a spice) or taken as a supplement. The supplements are generally considered safe but can interfere with blood clotting and should not be combined with any blood thinners (this includes aspirin and ibuprofen). Ginger can be used for fighting inflammation, but given in supplements it can be harmful, causing gallbladder issues and thinning of the blood. It is therefore our recommendation that ginger be consumed via dietary sources rather than taken as high-dose supplements. There are many great ways to use ginger in cooking, and it is a common ingredient in all forms of Asian cooking.

Arthritic complaints can be addressed with a number of supplements. In some cases they may not be a replacement for traditional medical therapy, but they can often be a useful addition to a treatment regimen. Similarly, a number of vitamins and supplements can play a role in addressing aches and pains related to muscle problems.

Vitamin D deficiency is notorious for causing both muscle aches and weakness (in addition to generalized fatigue and low bone density). In fact, in our practices we have seen several patients misdiagnosed as having severe neuromuscular conditions when they simply turned out to have low levels of vitamin D. Treating their deficiency with a vitamin D supplement reversed their symptoms. Correcting severe vitamin D deficiency does, however, require some time and patience, since vitamin D is a fat-soluble vitamin and it takes at least several months to build up your body stores. It is also recommended that vitamin D be taken with a high-fat meal for optimal absorption. We recommend taking its most active form, vitamin D3.

Another cause of muscle aches (or leg cramps) can be a magnesium deficiency. This essential electrolyte helps regulate channels that cause your muscle cells to contract and relax. Magnesium also is the gate-keeper for several other electrolytes, such as calcium and potassium. Without sufficient magnesium, your body cannot properly absorb and retain the other two electrolytes. Therefore, supplemental magnesium can be very helpful in preventing muscle cramps and aching.

People who take statin drugs (such as atorvastatin, simvastatin, pravastatin, etc.) to control cholesterol levels also can experience muscle aches. This symptom should be addressed with your doctor since there can be serious health consequences. However, it is most often just a short-lived discomfort that can sometimes be prevented by taking vitamin CoQ10 in conjunction with the cholesterol medicine. It is also our experience that patients who have optimal vitamin D levels are less prone to the side effects of these common medications.

It is important to consider that there are times when our muscles are more fatigued than others. Just as every person is not the same, each day is not the same. A big workout or a stressful day can tax our muscles more than usual. During those times, drinking lots of water and obtaining essential electrolytes and vitamins is key to put your muscles in an ideal position to work hard. Replenishing potassium, glucose, sodium chloride, and vitamin B12 (which is essential to energy and nerve function) is critical.

Taking supplemental electrolytes and B vitamins at specific times can help give you the boost by providing your muscles with the nutrients they need to function optimally and recover fast. We saw our patients over the years suffer from excess fatigue and achiness often after "overdoing it" with intense exercise or in less-than-ideal conditions, such as extreme heat. Once we realized that many of these symptoms could be avoided or remedied with the proper vitamins, our team at Vous Vitamin® created an ideal blend of electrolytes and B vitamins for working out, and called it Power Up™. Our customers love that they can take a tablet before and after exercise that is not filled with calories, sugar, and caffeine as many other electrolyte or energy products are.

We realize that the energy-drink market is vast and there are numerous products touted for their electrolyte replenishment.

However, it is our experience that many of these products are either high in calories or loaded up with artificial sweeteners and other chemicals. The more "natural" products, such as coconut water, do contain a decent amount of potassium and sodium, but often lack magnesium, chloride, and other key nutrients. They are also said to be an acquired taste. However, if you are in need of hydration, they are likely a better bet than plain water.

———————— ◆ ————————

A patient once said to us, "I hate the fact that when you are over fifty you wake up every morning and something new hurts. I guess it beats the alternative: not waking up." It doesn't have to be that bad!

Perhaps fifty actually is the new twenty, if you treat your body the way it deserves to be treated. Our patients who come in with these complaints find that by complementing their exercise preparation with the appropriate daily vitamin regimen, they feel young again. So, hydrate, make sure you are getting enough daily vitamins to meet your needs, and step it up when you need to with some extra electrolytes. With age we invariably take longer to recover from injury and are more prone to many musculoskeletal complaints, but we should not suffer in silence. We should Power Up™ and keep fighting the good fight. After careful consideration of the root origin of your discomfort—arthritic (joint related) or muscular—vitamins can be a part of the solution.

Most of us can take measures to improve how we feel at certain times. A thoughtful, measured, and comprehensive approach to treating aches and pains, as well as sniffles and coughs, can require a combination of lifestyle improvements and vitamins, which can help many of us feel better as we move forward.

CHAPTER 12
VITAMINS FOR PREGNANCY AND FERTILITY

WOMEN TODAY TYPICALLY START trying to conceive later in life than they did in past eras. Clearly many cultural and societal issues are behind this trend. With advancing age, the ability to easily get pregnant does decline for many women. However, infertility is an issue that plagues women (and men) of all ages. The good news is that we know more than ever about these issues and have a host of strategies at hand to help aid conception for those who want assistance in getting pregnant.

The field of medicine known as reproductive endocrinology has made incredible advances, some may argue almost to the point of science fiction–like capabilities. The ethical issues of reproductive technology are complicated and worthy of their own volume. However, we do encourage any woman with concerns about getting pregnant to seek medical advice early and often, since this is one aspect of health where the early bird does get the worm (the earlier in life you start trying, the higher your success rates typically are). That being said, not everyone needs high-tech interventions to conceive. There are some simple lifestyle and nutritional strategies, including the use of vitamins, that can enhance anyone's efforts to get pregnant.

So many women struggle with infertility issues. We hear so often the tales from women trying to conceive: counting each day of the month to determine ovulation, waiting on pins and needles to miss your period, wasting hundreds of dollars on home pregnancy tests, and the stress that can ensue from this process. Many common medical and nonmedical reasons may be the cause (do discuss these with your physician). Treatments from acupuncture to yoga to Chinese herbs have been tried with varying degrees of success. But perhaps first and foremost, getting a woman's own health in order is the biggest key to conception.

There are many factors included in optimal health, such as a healthful diet, regular exercise, sufficient sleep, a thorough gynecological checkup, and finding the right balance of certain nutrients. Good nutrition for the fetus is perhaps the first thing a woman can do to give her child a great start in life, even before conception, by adopting a complete and toxin-free diet (i.e., minimize processed foods).

However, some vitamins need supplementation since most people (even healthy eaters) do not get enough via diet alone. Getting the right vitamins before pregnancy is better for both getting pregnant and then having a healthy pregnancy and baby. And once a woman is pregnant, the role of vitamins in maintaining the pregnancy and optimizing the health of the mother and baby cannot be overstated.

We should make a distinction here between what is typically termed a "prenatal vitamin" and a typical multivitamin. The difference is actually often minimal and largely a matter of nomenclature. Of course products differ in their exact ingredients and amounts. But, generally speaking, a prenatal vitamin contains the typical multivitamin nutrients and is perhaps heavier on folic acid, iron, and iodine. Many common multivitamins, however, meet these needs adequately. The one component of prenatal regimens that is typically lacking in a multivitamin is the omega-3 component that is important later in pregnancy for neurological development. For this reason, most women can be well-served taking a traditional multivitamin up until conception. On the flip side, taking a prenatal vitamin for months leading up to conception is also perfectly acceptable and preferred to taking no vitamins at all. Many women take prenatal vitamins before, during, and after pregnancy.

At Vous Vitamin®, our latest wave of product development has focused on a prenatal booster to our Personalized Multivitamins™.

It was essential to us to find a way to add a high-quality omega-3 product to a vitamin regimen without compromising the purity of the product or the amounts needed to meet the standards of a quality prenatal product. In addition to containing other elements that are essential for pregnant women, this booster features a high-quality omega-3 product, which is an especially important component of any good prenatal vitamin.

A 2011 study in the United Kingdom showed that women taking a multivitamin were more likely to both get pregnant and stay pregnant. It is not surprising that getting adequate nutrition would be helpful in pregnancy. From an evolutionary standpoint it makes sense that women would be more likely to successfully carry a child if their own health needs are met adequately. We believe a few essential vitamins can be an important factor for most women who are trying to conceive.

Vitamin D deficiency is linked to infertility. Research shows women who have sufficient vitamin D levels are more likely to become pregnant (and produce high-quality embryos if undergoing in vitro) than those who are deficient in this essential vitamin. Somehow, we are not surprised. Vitamin D, more than other nutrients, has been found to be essential for things ranging from bone density to dementia prevention, immunity, and cancer prevention. It only makes sense that it would also play some role in fertility.

Vitamin D is a fat-soluble vitamin that we typically get from the sun. However, with the widespread use of sunscreen and the many of us who live in more temperate climates without year-round sun exposure, many or most of us have subnormal vitamin D levels. Because of the fat-soluble nature of vitamin D, it is slow to be absorbed and therefore can sometimes take six to twelve months to see levels normalize. (See other comments on the importance of vitamin D included in the Bone Health, Immunity, and Migraine chapters.)

Another vitamin that is important when trying to conceive is folate. This B vitamin plays a role in nerve growth and function. It is essential to fetal neural tube development. Women deficient in this when pregnant have higher risks of birth defects such as spina bifida (a sometimes severe spinal cord issue) in their babies.

While folate is found in many fruits and vegetables as well as some cereals and breads (which are fortified with it), it is generally recommended that women who are pregnant or trying to get pregnant take a supplement containing a form of folate, folic acid (starting at least six months in advance of trying to get pregnant). Many common multivitamins and prenatal vitamins contain significant amounts of this essential nutrient. However, many women do not realize that they should supplement in advance of trying to conceive. Most think only of taking prenatal vitamins once pregnant. Taking folic acid in advance of getting pregnant may help with both fertility itself and then the health of the fetus.

Similarly, when trying to get pregnant, it is important to have optimal thyroid function. The thyroid is a gland that regulates metabolism, and if not operating properly it is a common cause of infertility. The thyroid affects the brain's regulation of the menstrual cycle. Thus a woman whose thyroid is underactive may get erratic periods and not ovulate with regularity. Those who are prone to thyroid problems may need more or different medication when pregnant; thus, consult with your doctor prior to conception if at all possible. When it comes to vitamins, iodine plays an important role in thyroid function. The thyroid gland relies on iodine in proper amounts to produce thyroid hormone.

Worldwide, iodine deficiency is a huge problem and a significant cause of miscarriages and birth defects. In the Western world, many processed foods contain iodine due to their high iodized salt content. As many of us start eating more healthfully and avoiding processed foods, often cooking with sea salt or kosher salt, we have lost our source of iodine. Our attempts to be healthy have served us well in many regards but have failed us when it comes to iodine consumption and its role in thyroid health. Therefore, a good multivitamin should contain an adequate amount of iodine (but not an excess amount since that can have toxic effects). For pregnancy, the recommended amount of iodine increases to 220 mcg daily (and while nursing, more is required). While many of us get some of this from food sources, a supplement is often a good insurance policy. Many but not all prenatal vitamins contain the necessary iodine, so check yours to be certain it is included. But beware: Taking too much iodine can be dangerous, causing the thyroid to in fact malfunction. This is a situation where too much of a good thing is not better. (Read more on this in the Endocrinology and Metabolism chapter.)

Another vitamin that is important in conception, pregnancy, and the postpartum period is iron. Regular menstruation, pregnancy, and breastfeeding all are known to significantly deplete iron stores. It is best to get ahead of the game with an iron-containing vitamin. It is likely that building up iron stores is another way your body gets ready for conception. Once a woman is pregnant, the baby needs iron for development, and both mother and child rely on iron to make red blood cells that carry oxygen to tissues. However, many people have trouble with iron, which can cause an upset stomach or constipation.

We hear from many of our patients that they discontinue their prenatal vitamins because of GI symptoms. We have found that using the proper form of iron (such as carbonyl) in combination with the right balance of other nutrients can do the trick. It is also essential that the iron is paired with vitamin C for proper absorption. At Vous Vitamin®, we are very proud of the fact that a number of our customers report to us that they have never before been able to tolerate a multivitamin containing iron until they tried our Personalized Multivitamins™. We believe that using the proper dose, form, and combination of vitamins can make all the difference.

In addition to vitamins, many people try a variety of nontraditional means for conception. Yoga, acupuncture, and various Chinese herbs have all been touted as the non-Western secrets to fertility. We believe there is certainly a role for acupuncture and yoga. These two practices seem to help with relaxation, blood flow, and mental focus. If guided by well-trained professionals, they are not likely to cause harm and may be helpful. We are not advocates of Chinese herbs for this practice because we feel it is very difficult to know the source, purity, and safety of what you are taking. When trying to get pregnant, the last thing you want is to take something that could be toxic.

Thus, we believe traditional vitamins from a reputable source are preferred to less-known purveyors of herbal products.

The vitamins we have discussed thus far are all important parts of getting pregnant. In addition, each one of them is essential for maintaining a pregnancy and carrying a healthy baby. Vitamin D is likely as important for fetal development as it is for the health of our own adult cells. Folic acid's role in nerve function in adults is mirrored by its role in the neural tube formation of the fetus. Iodine's role in thyroid health is vital to getting pregnant, carrying a baby to term, and normal fetal development. Without it, babies are at risk for developmental delays and other birth defects. Iron is also essential to both a mother's health prior to conception and to supplying the baby with what it needs to thrive.

Another type of supplement that has become a routine part of prenatal care is omega-3 fatty acids, such as docosahexaenoic and eicosapentaenoic acids (DHA and EPA). This is due to some studies in the 2000s that show an association with fetal cognitive development and maternal DHA. Premature babies who get DHA supplements exhibit improvements in cognitive function and vision compared to those who do not get the supplements. There have also been studies that suggest some decline in premature birth and in postpartum depression among women taking omega-3s during pregnancy.

So many women find pregnancy a time when they start to really take their own health seriously. Many stop smoking and drinking alcohol for the benefit of their unborn child. These measures are wonderful and should not be overlooked. However, it is our plea to women everywhere who are not yet pregnant that they start thinking about their overall health prior to trying to conceive.

It is easier to focus on your health when you are not pregnant as you may be less tired and nauseated, and able to concentrate on your own diet and lifestyle choices. Entering this phase of life in optimal health, you will likely get pregnant more easily, have a healthy full-term pregnancy, and produce a thriving baby by getting a head start on the proper nutrients before your body undergoes the stress of pregnancy. In short, it's never too early (or too late, for that matter) to start laying the proper groundwork with diet, exercise, and nutritional supplements for childbearing.

PART THREE: VITAMINS FOR PREVENTION

CHAPTER 13
SLEEP

NO DISCUSSION OF GOOD HEALTH is complete without addressing sleep. This vital bodily function is so very essential to just about every other aspect of our well-being that we almost always review sleep patterns with our patients. There are many things most of us can do to improve our sleep quality and duration, and vitamins and supplements can play a significant role in optimizing these sleep habits. In theory we should all be spending about one third of our time sleeping, so let us touch on how and why to best make good sleep part of your routine.

First off, let's touch on what can happen if you don't sleep enough: bad things. Lots of them. The seemingly harmless habit of shaving off an hour here and there (perhaps to get up early for work or because you have trouble getting to sleep) can ultimately have major consequences. Lack of sleep correlates with the development of and worsening of many chronic health conditions. The best examples of how lack of sleep can lead to illness come from research on common sleep disorders.

Sleep disorders such as sleep apnea have been linked directly to conditions such as obesity, heart failure, high blood pressure, diabetes, depression, fibromyalgia, and more. In fact, people with severe untreated sleep apnea are actually twice as likely to die prematurely as people who do not have it. You get the picture.

In recent years we have found that optimizing sleep can in fact help treat many of the above-listed conditions. For many people it may not be as simple as spending more time in bed. Diagnosing and treating sleep apnea is something that must be done by a trained medical professional. Treating this condition can help reverse many of the aforementioned associated conditions.

However, even if sleep apnea is not a concern, we commonly advise our patients who struggle with weight loss to make sure they are getting enough sleep. So, just sleep more to lose weight! Seems too good to be true, right?

Sleeping too little can in fact promote weight gain, and this may be your worst nightmare! Studies have shown that sleep is in fact inextricably related to weight, because several hormones that your body produces while you sleep, such as ghrelin and leptin, regulate weight and appetite control; and hormones cannot be produced properly with fewer than seven hours of sleep. Research has also shown that people who are sleep deprived tend to crave higher-calorie foods. When you are tired, you are also less motivated to exercise and make the effort it takes to eat a healthful diet. It's easy to see how the pounds pile on.

In addition to major medical issues, the obvious result of not enough sleep is lack of energy or fatigue. (See the Energy and Fatigue chapter for more ways to address this problem.) When it comes to fatigue, there is no replacement for sleeping long enough and well enough. How much is enough? Well, as you've heard before, we are all different. We each have a different ideal amount of sleep. However, in general it tends to be more than you think. Some experts say seven to nine hours is sufficient for most adults, while some women may need up to ten hours per night. A small minority of people need significantly less sleep than that. Some überproductive examples are Martha Stewart and Bill Clinton.

Another factor to consider is the issue of quality of sleep. Even if you are in bed sleeping for a reasonable period of time, the eight hours may be interrupted hours or not "good" sleep. Your body may never be reaching the stages of deep restorative sleep it needs to function at its best. The reasons for poor sleep may include sleep apnea, snoring, restless leg syndrome, and other sleep disturbances attributable to medical causes and external ones (for example, children). If you suspect that you are getting a sufficient amount of sleep but are still tired, you might consider consulting with your physician about testing for various sleep disorders.

Here's one more catch: if you are behind in your sleep, you accumulate a sleep debt—a deficit of sleep that you need to replenish. So sleeping in on the weekend is not going to make up for day after day of sleep deprivation. You actually need to make up those lost hours. That sleep-deprived mother of a newborn may need years—yes, *years*—to recover from all those months of sleeplessness, even once her kids are sleeping through the night. So if you are chronically sleep deprived, you best get to bed now and start making up for lost time!

However, sleep isn't always easy to come by, even if you are dedicated to the cause. Some tips for getting to sleep:

- Have a regular bedtime and wake-up time. This helps your internal clock and circadian rhythms stay consistent. Forcing yourself to wake up at a consistent time will be the best way to get yourself to sleep at a reasonable hour.

- Stop all caffeine consumption at noon. Believe it or not, its effects last way longer than you think.

- Minimize alcohol (more on this later). While you think it makes you fall asleep, ultimately it disrupts your ability to get good-quality sleep.

- Stop screen time at least an hour before bedtime. Yes, that means reading an old-fashioned book. You know, the paper kind. Screens (especially phone or iPad screens that are close to your eyes) signal to your brain it's time to wake up.

- Make sure your room is dark, comfortable, and on the cool side.

- Make your bed a place just for sleeping. Don't associate with wake-time activities (TV, work, etc.).

- Try calming foods prior to bedtime, such as chamomile tea or warm milk.

- Take a warm bath to relax.

- Avoid exercise for three hours prior to bedtime. (However, regular exercise earlier in the day is great for nighttime sleep.)

- Avoid naps longer than fifteen or twenty minutes. Sometimes a little afternoon snooze can hit the spot. Many progressive companies now feature nap rooms for their employees because of the boost in productivity that results. However, don't overdo it since too much sleep during the day will come back to bite you at bedtime.

- Try a common relaxation technique, such as guided meditation or yogic breathing, or clear your mind by counting backwards from 400 in intervals of four. One expert recommends that you "focus on looking at the inside of your eyes." All of these options seek to shift your attention from running to-do lists or the litany of thoughts running through your head.

Vitamins You Can't Sleep Without

As with many other aspects of our health, the right vitamins play a key role in good sleep habits. Deficiencies in certain areas can range from subtle effects on sleep to profound disturbances. There may be an insidious onset over many years or a dramatic sign that seems to show up all of sudden. Either way, it is important to consider the following nutrients and how supplementing them may help your struggles with sleep.

IRON

We all know iron is important for energy. However, few people realize that being iron deficient not only makes you feel tired, but can actually make you more likely to have a condition called Restless Leg Syndrome. People with this condition have constant movement and twitching sensations in their legs just when they are trying to fall asleep.

Many of us have unrecognized iron deficiency that does not come up in typical blood counts. Low iron stores can be repleted with the proper vitamins to address this. Correcting iron deficiency can also help make restless legs disappear and stop sabotaging your sleep.

MELATONIN

This is known as the essential sleep vitamin. Actually it's a hormone that our brains typically manufacture to tell our bodies when to sleep. When our natural sleep rhythms get disturbed (such as via jet lag or an altered schedule of staying up too late) melatonin can be used to get us back on track.

Taking this natural supplement, typically 1–5 mg (make sure to get a reputable brand to ensure quality and purity) about thirty minutes before bed, helps to naturally reset your body's clock so you essentially relearn when bedtime should be.

MAGNESIUM

As we've mentioned in other chapters, magnesium is essential to making all of our cells function properly. Its role in sleep is likely dual. It may help with the actual mechanism by which our brain relaxes to fall asleep (by stimulating GABA receptors). It is also essential for helping with muscle cramps that are a common cause of a poor night's sleep.

Correcting magnesium deficiency helps your body with the natural process of falling asleep and at the same time can rid you of those painful muscle cramps. Magnesium is an electrolyte we can't live without and certainly can't sleep (well) without.

VITAMIN B12

People who are deficient in vitamin B12 (common among vegetarians or vegans, or those regularly taking medications for acid reflux) often experience what is called neuropathy. These are sensations of tingling or burning pain in the feet or hands. The symptoms of B12 deficiency are typically worse at night and are quick to ruin a night's sleep. B12 deficiency can also interfere with memory and cognition. Correcting a B12 deficiency can help get rid of these annoying symptoms and leave you free to rest.

VITAMIN D

The more we learn about this important vitamin, the more we love it. We find it plays a role in many facets of our health, sleep included. We know that without enough vitamin D, many of us experience muscle aches and fatigue. Of course, both of these things can relate to sleep—muscle aches limiting our ability to sleep and fatigue causing us to want more sleep. More and more research suggests that there is a strong correlation between lack of sleep and insufficient amounts of vitamin D. This is an easy one to correct with the proper dose of a supplement.

BLACK COHOSH

This herb may be your best friend if you are not sleeping well because of menopausal symptoms. Hot flashes are a huge disrupter of sleep (whether you are conscious of them or not). For this reason, many women find that with menopause come daytime fatigue, weight gain, irritability, and other hallmarks of sleep deprivation. (See the chapter on Menopause for more potential treatment strategies for the pesky symptoms that can accompany this phase of life.) Black cohosh is an herb commonly touted for helping reduce hot-flash frequency and symptoms. For some it is supremely helpful, for others not so much. It may come in handy in your quest for better, less interrupted sleep.

———————•◆•———————

In summary, sleep seems like such a simple thing, but it is in fact the confluence of many important things coming together just so in order to keep your body functioning at its best during waking hours. Most of us do not give it the priority we should, but it is never too late to start.

As physicians, we often hear dramatic stories from our patients with sleep apnea who have essentially lived in a chronic state of sleep deprivation. Once treated successfully (usually with an apparatus they wear during sleep that facilitates breathing while asleep) many people are in a sense reborn. They experience life completely differently in a rested state. Many are able to lose the weight they struggled to shed before. In addition, their chronic medical problems often improve drastically.

Some of us may be struggling with these issues on a lower level. Vitamin deficiencies, sleep hygiene, and lifestyle factors are all things to consider in your personal journey to a well-rested state. Pleasant dreams!

CHAPTER 14
BONE HEALTH

IT IS TEMPTING TO THINK of bones as fixed, finished products in our body. However, quite the opposite is true. Our bones are constantly remodeling. They contain living cells that continually absorb minerals to replace old, dead cells. In the process, old bone is broken down and new bone is built. This is both good and bad news. The good news: Because new bone can be built at any time, there are always opportunities to build up your bones. The bad news: Building new bone requires a constant source of the right minerals (namely calcium and phosphorus) to create the new bone.

It is important to understand that there is a continual opposition between bone breakdown and bone growth. Early in our lives, the bone-building forces win out and we gain bone density throughout childhood, adolescence, and young adulthood. Our bone density tends to peak around age thirty-five, and then, as with many other things in our bodies, it's all downhill from there as the bones slowly start to break down and thin—once a threshold in low bone density is crossed, osteopenia is diagnosed; and when a critical point in low bone density is reached, it is known as osteoporosis.

Women's bone density tends to take a particularly big dive after we hit menopause (because we lose all the estrogen that helps maintain bone density). As this bone breakdown progresses, our bones lose their density (or mineralization) and we become vulnerable to fragility fractures—broken bones related to low bone density and the brittle nature of demineralized bones. The most common such problems are hip fractures, broken wrists, and vertebral fractures (painful compression of the spine bones that can ultimately lead to a loss of height or a humpbacked appearance—think hunched-over old woman).

Fractures due to osteoporosis can be painful, debilitating, and, especially in the case of broken hips, even deadly. Hip fractures are associated with a high short-term and longer-term mortality and are often fraught with complications such as pneumonia and blood clots. In fact, some studies show that women with a hip fracture have twice as high a death rate in the year following the break. For this reason, bone density is a silent killer. Many people do not realize they have osteoporosis until they sustain a fracture.

But wait—it's not really that bad! Even though these bone-breakdown forces dominate as we age, there are still things we can do to delay or slow down the process. So it only makes sense to try to prevent all of this. The more we do earlier in life, the better off we will be as we age. However, intervention at any stage in bone health can make a difference.

Let's first look at who is more at risk.

As we mentioned, women generally get a raw deal when it comes to bones. We are all at significant risk for osteoporosis, especially now that our life expectancy is so long. Men have testosterone that helps them much of their lives with bone strength; but for women, the estrogen that helps protect our bones (and tips the balance toward building bone density) drops off severely when we hit menopause. Not surprisingly, women who do not have sufficient estrogen earlier in life are at higher risk. The typical causes for this are women who do not get regular menstrual periods, such as those with eating disorders, extreme exercise regimens that cause menstruation to stop, or other hormonal problems (polycystic ovary syndrome, for example). These are topics to discuss with your doctor if they affect you; birth control pills are often prescribed for these women because of the estrogen they contain.

Among women with normal periods during their younger lives, those who enter menopause early will then naturally start the decline in bone density early. The average age is fifty, but the earlier you stop getting your period, the more at risk you are.

Other risk factors for developing osteoporosis include the following:

- low body weight or small frame
- history of a fragility fracture
- parental history of a hip fracture
- long-term use of oral steroids (such as prednisone for diseases like asthma or rheumatoid arthritis)
- smoking
- drinking more than three alcoholic drinks daily
- hyperthyroidism (from an overactive thyroid or taking too much thyroid replacement)
- GI conditions such as celiac and Crohn's, or having had intestinal bypass surgery

How do we determine who has low bone density? The current standard of care for bone density testing is the DEXA (dual-energy X-ray absorptiometry) scan. (See the Screening Tests chapter for more on who should have this test done and when; the scan does not provide helpful information unless it is performed in the correct setting.)

Whether you know you already have low bone density or you are aiming to prevent it, there are many simple lifestyle changes that can be effective. However, it is important to remember that losing bone density is a slow process that occurs over many, many years. (As we like to say, there is no such thing as a bone density emergency.) The flip side of this is that preventing or reversing bone density are also slow, long-haul processes that take decades to work. Every day does count, so there's no time like the present to get started!

How do we go about avoiding the progressive loss of bone density? The most common way to address it, and the thing that is important at any age, is to make sure you provide your bones with the proper building blocks so they can build up strength. Namely, that is calcium. Sounds simple? Well it's not. At least if you watch the news it sounds

awfully complicated. The bottom line is there has been a lot of controversy over the last few years about who should take calcium and
how much.

The Calcium Conversation

Getting enough calcium is useful in building bone density. If calcium
prevents osteoporosis, it makes sense that eating things with calcium
and taking a supplement with calcium is a good idea. So taking more
supplements is probably better, right? Well, that was the thought. . .
Until recently, we were in fact doling out calcium supplements for
women as if they were candy. The intention was good: Calcium builds
bones. Bone density declines with age, so as women are living longer,
osteoporosis has reached epidemic proportions. Therefore, it makes
sense that we should do anything we can to prevent or minimize this
troublesome condition. But is there such a thing as too much calcium?

Our previous recommendations included calcium supplements of
1,200–1,500 mg per day. The highest doses were for older women or
those with known bone loss. These supplements usually come in the
form of large, difficult-to-swallow tablets that were supposed to be
taken multiple times daily with food (for better absorption). Beyond the
hassle factor, other downsides to taking calcium supplements include
unwanted side effects such as upset stomach, kidney stones, constipation, interference with other drugs, and, less commonly, serious
overdoses with high blood levels of calcium (which can even lead to
coma). All of that aside, more than half of older women in the United
States are still taking these supplements in the name of bone density.

However, it turns out that taking calcium supplements may also
cause unintended harm, particularly when one ingests large amounts,
as the calcium may not just make its way to your bones but could also
deposit itself in other places in your body—of greatest concern are
the important blood vessels that supply your heart and your brain.
That's right, all this circulating calcium may actually clog your
arteries and contribute to heart disease and stroke. But wait—we
aren't sounding the alarm bells yet, because the data still is not definitive and continue to be tested. In fact, a large study in 2014 disputed

this theory, showing that a large group of women taking supplements did not have a greater risk of these problems.

In our medical opinion, the sensible solution to preserving your bones is to avoid megadoses of calcium supplements for now, but to remember that dietary calcium still is important. As with most vitamins, it is always best to obtain nutrients from food rather than pills. We believe that with few exceptions most people can get a significant amount of their needed calcium from what they eat. It can however take a little effort and planning.

The current National Osteoporosis Foundation guidelines recommend 1,000 mg of calcium for women up to age fifty and men up to age seventy. Over those ages, they advise 1,200 mg daily. As you start looking at foods to determine their calcium content, one tip on label reading: The U.S. daily value (DV) for calcium—i.e., their recommended daily intake that does not take into consideration age, sex, and health history—is 1,000 mg. Therefore, percentage of DV given can be equated with milligrams as such: Something that is 30 percent of DV is 300 mg, 20 percent of DV is 200 mg, and so forth. You can use this to do a quick tally of your daily intake.

There are many great sources from which you can get your daily calcium in addition to the commonly thought of milk, cheese, and yogurt (see table below). These dairy sources are the best bang for your buck in terms of calcium. Greek yogurt leads the pack. We advise our patients that if you enjoy yogurt, having one a day is a great start for your daily calcium intake. Many of the Greek yogurts, save those filled with too much added sugar, are a sensible breakfast option since they also contain a nice protein serving. (See more about this benefit in the Nutrition and Weight Loss chapters.)

Contrary to popular belief, however, dairy is not the only way to get calcium, so vegans or individuals with lactose intolerance need not despair. Green leafy vegetables such as kale, spinach, watercress, and broccoli, or even nuts and seeds such as sesame seeds, almonds, and chickpeas are all good sources. Many of the nondairy milk options (almond, rice, and soy) also contain good amounts of calcium, as do some fortified foods, namely orange juice, tofu, and some breads.

With all of these options and a bit of planning, most of us can cobble together at least 1,000 mg or so daily via all of these food sources.

All of that said, many of us may still need to take a small amount of calcium supplement to reach our 1,000 mg or 1,200 mg daily goal. But gone are the days of the big calcium pills. Each person should find the right amount of supplement for his or her individual needs (the big milk drinker may need less than the lactose-intolerant person, for example). See the table below for some common foods and their calcium contents. Supplemental calcium comes in many forms, including tablets, candies, chews, and even some antacids (such as Tums®). The most common forms of calcium supplements are carbonate and gluconate. Both are useful and effective, though it is commonly warned that calcium carbonate is better absorbed if taken with food. Some find calcium citrate less likely to cause constipation and this formulation does not need to be taken with food. It is also important to remember that the GI tract can only absorb so much calcium at a time (probably 500 mg maximum). Therefore, if you take a supplement, it should not be taken at the same time as other high-calcium foods. Better to spread these sources out throughout the day.

Vitamin D

No discussion of building bone density would be complete without mention of vitamin D. This often-overlooked vitamin is high on our hit list of important vitamins. You will read about it in many other chapters in this book (as it pertains to energy, thinning hair, muscle aches, and other ailments). In the context of bone density, vitamin D is essential for proper calcium absorption. In fact, our entire discussion of calcium intake is irrelevant if you do not have enough vitamin D to absorb the calcium. And guess what? Many of us do not have enough vitamin D.

Historically, people have gotten vitamin D from the sun, but, depending on where you live, many people do not get enough year-round sun exposure to sustain a high enough vitamin D level. Additionally, sun protection measures such as sunscreen further compromise our exposure (and sun protection should be employed since it is our best way to avoid skin cancer). As we get older we do not absorb and metabolize vitamin D from the sun adequately. We see many patients in our Midwestern practice who spend the winter in Florida or Arizona, getting generous sun exposure. Rarely are their vitamin D levels adequate. The take-home is that most of us do need supplemental vitamin D for bone health. It should be taken in its most active form, D3, from a quality source. It is best taken with food for adequate absorption.

The amount of vitamin D to take varies based on several factors—namely where you live and if you are at risk for not absorbing it orally (having IBD or other conditions). Blood levels can be helpful in assessing vitamin D levels but are not mandatory. Taking a moderate supplemental dose (usually 800–2,000 IU daily) is not likely to cause harm (as some much higher doses can, refer to Vitamin Horror Stories).

Other Vitamins for Bone Health

One less commonly mentioned vitamin that is likely to play a role in bone health is magnesium. Several studies show that taking supplemental magnesium is helpful in bone density. This makes sense since magnesium is stored in bones and plays a role in vitamin D regulation as well as bone turnover. Taking some supplemental magnesium (approximately 300 mg daily) is likely a good idea and rarely causes harm. Only people with kidney disease are at risk for problems from taking this low a dose of magnesium.

There is discussion among many naturopathic sources about the role of vitamin K—or specifically one component thereof, vitamin K2—in bone health. At this time we do not see sufficient medical evidence to support using vitamin K supplements for bone health. Few of us are deficient in vitamin K. It is in fact one of the only vitamins our body produces naturally (bacteria in our colon actually make it). More studies are sure to be done to flesh out the role of vitamin K in bone health, but the studies that have been done so far have been conflicting and lacking in evidence regarding its usefulness in this area, so stay tuned on this one.

Exercise

As we've described, bones are living, evolving cells that respond to not only the nutrients put before them but also to certain environmental influences. Namely, applying pressure to bones or "weight-bearing" activities actually causes the bones to respond by becoming stronger. It's not dissimilar to the idea of using weight lifting to grow your muscles. This is why larger framed and overweight people are generally at lower risk for low bone density; the weight they carry around on a daily basis actually helps build their bones. Those who have slighter frames and less body mass have less resistance on a regular basis to keep nudging their bones to strengthen. To be clear, we are not telling you to gain weight to build your bone strength. This can actually be achieved by doing proper weight-bearing exercises. Routinely putting pressure on your bones will help increase bone density. The good news is that most exercise is weight bearing in some way. You can enhance the upper-body effect of using an elliptical or walking by using your arms more vigorously and adding one-pound wrist weights (these can be purchased at any local fitness store, or Target, or Wal-Mart).

The one exercise that does not really "count" as weight bearing (though it is a good calorie burn) is swimming. The water reduces resistance so your bones don't get the pressure they need to promote bone density. However, some people do water-aerobics classes that use light weights, and these *do* qualify as weight bearing.

In addition to weight bearing for the sake of strengthening bones, strength training and balance training are great for those with low bone density. Not only do strength and balance training help build bones themselves, but they inherently help with fall prevention. Activities like yoga, martial arts, and tai chi are great ways to get exercise that strengthens bones and at the same times teaches balance techniques that will in turn help prevent falls and fractures.

Other Treatments

Patients with an established diagnosis of osteoporosis or osteopenia (lower-grade bone loss) have numerous prescription treatment options, though these options are highly individualistic and necessitate a discussion with your physician. Especially in cases of osteopenia, a tool called the Fracture Risk Assessment Tool (FRAX®) score should be employed to determine the likelihood that an individual will sustain a fracture. If the likelihood of a fracture in the next ten years is high enough (experts say 3 percent for a hip fracture or 20 percent for a nonhip fragility fracture), guidelines advise treatment with a bisphosphonate. These drugs—the most common of which is Fosamax®—have received somewhat of a bad rap over the years. Lots of lay press has enjoyed touting their nasty side effects. They certainly can have associated side effects—the most common and untoward of which is GI and esophageal symptoms—so they should be taken on an empty stomach accompanied by a full glass of water, and you must remain upright (not lying down) for thirty minutes to an hour after taking them and not eat during this time. So it's a bit of an ordeal, but there are once-weekly or once-monthly doses available that help most people find it doable.

Bisphosphonates' much rarer and dreaded complication of "osteo-necrosis of the jaw" is often talked about but almost never seen (it occurs in one in a quarter of a million people or fewer who take bisphosphonates). The majority of cases have been seen in patients who are receiving higher-than-typical doses for specific cancer conditions. In most, it can be avoided if you obtain good dental care and stop the medication around times of tooth extractions. Check with your dentist on this one.

Another headline about bisphosphonates relates to fractures said to be caused by these treatments for osteoporosis. Further examination of these atypical types of femur fractures has revealed that they typically occur in people who have osteoporosis associated only with long-term steroid (prednisone) use. People with osteoporosis due to chronic steroid use may benefit from another type of treatment.

A final word on osteoporosis treatment and prevention, and the role of HRT. At one time, it was standard to put women automatically on hormones when they hit menopause. There is no doubt that hormone replacement (the estrogen component) does strengthen bones and essentially slow the normal postmenopausal decline. However, this is no longer considered enough of a reason to start HRT. It may be a factor in a decision, but there are too many potential negatives to using HRT (increased rates of breast cancer, stroke, and cardiac disease) to endorse using it for bone density alone. That being said, for some women with specific circumstances or conditions, HRT is the correct choice and bone density will likely benefit. This is a conversation to have with your physician since it is such an individual decision. Do note that "compounded" or non-FDA-approved treatments for menopausal symptoms, commonly called "bioidenticals," have not been sufficiently tested for their role in treating bone density, or any other conditions, nor have they been tested sufficiently to be considered safe in anyone.

In addition to those we have discussed here, there are a number of other prescription treatments for osteoporosis. These medications are beyond the scope of this book, but suffice it to say, there are a whole host of options for treating bone density today, most of which did not exist fifteen years ago. Bone density is a slow-to-change condition, but that does not mean it should be ignored. Be sure to have a discussion with your physician about what treatment may be best suited to your needs.

CALCIUM-RICH FOODS

FOOD	MILLIGRAMS (MG) PER SERVING	PERCENT DV*
Yogurt, plain, low fat, 8 ounces	415	42
Mozzarella, part skim, 1.5 ounces	333	33
Sardines, canned in oil, with bones, 3 ounces	325	33
Yogurt, fruit, low fat, 8 ounces	313–384	31–38
Cheese, cheddar, 1.5 ounces	307	31
Milk, nonfat, 8 ounces**	299	30
Soymilk, calcium-fortified, 8 ounces	299	30
Milk, reduced fat (2% milk fat), 8 ounces	293	29

Milk, buttermilk, low fat, 8 ounces	284	28
Milk, whole (3.25% milk fat), 8 ounces	276	28
Orange juice, calcium-fortified, 6 ounces	261	26
Tofu, firm, made with calcium sulfate, ½ cup***	253	25
Salmon, pink, canned, solids with bone, 3 ounces	181	18
Cheese, cottage, 1% milk fat, 1 cup	138	14
Tofu, soft, made with calcium sulfate, ½ cup***	138	14
Cereal, ready to eat, calcium fortified, 1 cup	100–1,000	10–100
Frozen yogurt, vanilla, soft serve, ½ cup	103	10
Turnip greens, fresh, boiled, ½ cup	99	10
Kale, raw, chopped, 1 cup	100	10
Kale, fresh, cooked, 1 cup	94	9
Ice cream, vanilla, ½ cup	84	8
Chinese cabbage, bok choy, raw, shredded, 1 cup	74	7
Bread, white, 1 slice	73	7
Pudding, chocolate, ready to eat, refrigerated, 4 ounces	55	6
Tortilla, corn, ready to bake/fry, one 6-inch diameter	46	5
Tortilla, flour, ready to bake/fry, one 6-inch diameter	32	3
Sour cream, reduced fat, cultured, 2 tablespoons	31	3
Bread, whole wheat, 1 slice	30	3
Broccoli, raw, ½ cup	21	2
Cheese, cream, regular, 1 tablespoon	14	1

* DV = Daily Value. DVs were developed by the U.S. Food and Drug Administration (FDA) to help consumers compare the nutrient contents among products within the context of a total daily diet. The DV for calcium is 1,000 mg for adults and children aged four years and older. Foods providing 20% or more of the DV are considered to be high sources of a nutrient, but foods providing lower percentages of the DV also contribute to a healthful diet. The U.S. Department of Agriculture's (USDA) Nutrient Database Web site lists the nutrient content of many foods and provides a comprehensive list of foods containing calcium arranged by nutrient content and by food name.

** Calcium content varies slightly by fat content; typically the more fat, the less calcium the food contains.

*** Calcium content is for tofu processed with a calcium salt. Tofu processed with other salts does not provide significant amounts of calcium.

CHAPTER 15
MEMORY AND ATTENTION

CONCERNS ABOUT MEMORY LOSS ABOUND. As our population ages, we see people all around us suffering from various forms of cognitive decline. Those of us who are not yet in the age group typical for Alzheimer's and other forms of dementia are still concerned because we want to know how to prevent memory loss. As physicians, one of the most common questions we hear is, "What vitamins can I take for memory and concentration?"

Firstly, let us touch on the relationship between memory and concentration (or attention). They are clearly very different issues—memory concerns recalling information and facts, while concentration refers to the ability to focus on something. While memory and concentration are distinct measures, they are forever intertwined because without the ability to concentrate and attend to something, you cannot focus enough to remember facts. Both abilities are related to brain and neurological function. Not surprisingly then, many of the vitamins involved address both of these issues simultaneously.

It seems that everyone either suffers from problems with memory or is concerned about developing them. And they should be. Recent data shows that nearly one third of Americans over the age of seventy have some form of memory problem. As people are living to older ages due to great treatment breakthroughs in heart disease and cancer, they are sticking around longer in body, but their minds often decline.

Yet we hear complaints about memory trouble from people even in their thirties and forties. It is our experience that these people suffer more from a concentration issue than a memory issue. They tend to multitask to the nth degree, and this interferes with their ability to remember things. If you are doing too many things at once, it is very hard to either retain new information or recall old information. This problem seems to be on the upswing as mobile devices further infiltrate so many aspects of our lives. We are rarely focusing on any one thing enough to really have full recall or to create solid memories.

While memory trouble and attention issues are similar in many ways and can in fact be related, they are by no means the same problem. Thus we will delve into the issue that seems to plague more of us in our younger years first, attention, and then move into one of our country's greatest issues as our population ages, memory. Oh wait . . . did we say that already?

Vitamins for Attention

Distractions aside, we often hear about the diagnosis of attention deficit disorder (ADD). This term is used to describe both children and adults who have an impaired ability to stay on task. As with most diagnoses, it encompasses a spectrum of traits, which can manifest in different ways in different people. Not surprisingly, people's response to different treatments also varies greatly from person to person. There is a huge range of treatment options; some are doctor-prescribed and others are vitamins and supplements. This is, of course, in addition to many behavioral techniques that can and should be tried.

The diagnosis of ADD seems to come readily these days. Going into all its nuances is best left to psychiatrists and other experts in that field as are the various prescription medications. Suffice it to say, sometimes we believe medication is doled out too easily, and there are major downsides to many of the commonly used stimulants. Not only can they be addictive, but they can have dangerous side effects, particularly involving blood pressure and cardiac effects. Needless to say, they should only be used when absolutely necessary. Sometimes vitamins can help to minimize the dose of medication needed or avoid it all together.

Of all the supplements touted for attention, omega-3s (typically found as fish oil) are probably the most studied in this context. Data

suggests that regular use of them can improve attention in both children and adults. EPA and DHA seem to play some role in brain
development and are also found in prenatal supplements and baby
formula for this reason. How much to take still seems up for debate,
though standard dosing is generally about 1,000 mg daily of a
combined EPA/DHA supplement.

Magnesium has also been suggested to be helpful for ADD. Groups
of children studied showed less hyperactivity when given magnesium
supplements. It seems that these findings might carry over to adults
struggling to attend to various tasks but has yet been established.
Magnesium's important role in cellular function throughout the body
may help with attention by improving the function of nerve cells.

Some have suggested zinc can be useful to attention, however data
is fairly inconclusive. In our opinion, heavy metals should not be taken
in supplements regularly unless there is a compelling reason. We do
not believe that the evidence supports taking zinc daily for attention.

In the late '90s and early 2000s, St. John's wort was all the rage
for many conditions. It was suggested to play a useful role in attention,
but this has not been borne out by scientific findings. In fact, many
studies do not support its use for this purpose. We also advise extreme
caution in using this herb since it has many potential interactions with
other medications and side effects (including extreme reactions such
as psychosis—or a dissociation with reality).

We would be remiss if we did not mention caffeine in a discussion of attention. It is known by everyone from high school-aged
kids on up that caffeine helps with attention and concentration. The
"energy" market is thriving and chock-full of products loaded with
caffeine, promoted for their ability to enhance academic and/or
athletic performance. There is some basis for this. Caffeine works.
However, as mentioned in the Weight Loss chapter, we believe
strongly that caffeine should be obtained in moderate amounts from
natural sources such as coffee or tea. The use of caffeine products
and supplements can be both highly dangerous and ineffective (since
high doses can often backfire and cause such a rush of energy that
people experience anxiety and an inability to function). Overuse

also interferes with sleep, which can really come back to bite you the next day.

The aforementioned vitamins have been suggested as useful for attention. However, one of the most commonly used supplements for ADD is melatonin. It is not used for the attention issue itself but rather to combat the insomnia that often accompanies prescription medication for ADD (stimulants). The use of melatonin is fairly widespread in both children and adults (see more in our chapter on sleep) and is generally considered safe and effective, though the wide range of dosing (typically between 1 and 15 mg nightly) sometimes requires trial and error to determine the ideal amount for each person.

Vitamins for Memory

While trouble attending to the task at hand may plague many of us in our earlier years, the complaints seem to shift starting in our fifties to concerns about memory. As we mentioned previously, the two are integrally related. However, the aging population has a much higher incidence of Alzheimer's disease and other types of dementia (progressive loss of memory cognitive abilities), and it increases with each decade of age. As the population as a whole ages, at a minimum we can expect a whole lot of people wandering around parking lots having forgotten where they parked their cars.

Since many of us have been touched by this problem through a family member or otherwise, trying to prevent dementia is on the forefront of many people's list of concerns. Experts have put out many recommendations about lifestyle factors that can lead to lower rates of dementia. These typically include things that comprise a generally healthy lifestyle, such as regular exercise, moderate alcohol intake, good sleep habits, and a diet high in fruits, vegetables, and whole grains and low in fats and sugars. In addition, keeping your brain active with things like crossword puzzles, Sudoku, and regular social interactions are also known to help with the continued firing of those brain cells.

However, many people would like to go beyond lifestyle changes to prevent memory loss. It is certainly worth considering what vitamins or supplements to take for memory loss and concentration. There is a great deal of research out there about many different vitamins for memory, but limited evidence showing some conclusive proof that these vitamins prevent memory loss.

First, there are the B vitamins for memory. It has been clearly established that people who are low in vitamin B12 have a number of neurological issues. Included in the symptoms of B12 deficiency are memory loss and low energy, among other things. Arielle has seen patients over the years who have come in with significant concerns about memory and/or attention (people ranging in age from college students to the elderly); and upon further analysis of their diet and health, she has found they are profoundly B12 deficient. Correction of this deficiency can work wonders. Replacing B12 either through oral daily doses or, occasionally, high-dose injections (discuss with your doctor) or prescription nasal preparations can improve these symptoms. B12 is an established vitamin that helps with memory and brain function in those who need it.

People who rarely eat meat are often low in this important vitamin. However, it remains unclear whether taking this B vitamin helps memory in someone who does not have a deficiency. One smaller study showed some improvement in memory and cognition in people taking a combination of vitamin B12 and folic acid.

B6 is another vitamin for dementia prevention that showed some promising effects when combined with B12 and folic acid. Another study showed some delay in onset of memory loss in those taking these vitamins for dementia. We conclude that these vitamins are potentially helpful as B12, B6, and folic acid are essential for brain and nerve function. There is little downside to taking them in appropriate doses.

Other research about vitamins for memory loss has included some data on antioxidant vitamins such as vitamins C and E. There is some conflicting data but enough information to suggest that reasonable doses of these vitamins may help prevent memory loss. They seem to protect against vascular dementia (related to small strokes) more so than Alzheimer's-type dementia. However, many people with memory loss have features of both types of diseases, so helping the vascular component would be useful. Vitamins C and E seem to help prevent dementia because they have an anticoagulant or blood-thinning effect. For this reason, they should only be taken in moderate doses and with caution in someone who has a risk of bleeding.

Perhaps one of the most compelling bits of recent research in regard to vitamins for memory and cognition is that regarding vitamin D. Vitamin D is one of the most important vitamins we recommend. You have heard us wax poetic about its usefulness for bone health, general well-being, energy, and immunity. A 2014 study looked at people with different blood levels of vitamin D and found that those with very low levels of vitamin D were about 50 percent more likely to develop dementia. From this, one can conclude that raising vitamin D levels may help prevent memory loss, though it has not yet been proven. It is known that vitamin D may play a role in inflammation in the brain, and this inflammation could be part of why people lose memory. We conclude that for this, among many other reasons, taking supplemental vitamin D to prevent memory loss is important.

Another consideration when trying to prevent memory loss with vitamins is supplements for memory loss derived from natural plants such as turmeric. Turmeric, also known as curcumin, is a spice used frequently in Indian cooking and curries. This flavorful yellow powder may have benefits in preventing inflammatory processes including Alzheimer's disease. It was first noted that the people of India have much lower rates of dementia than their Western counterparts. Then several studies were done showing improvement in parts of the brain affected by Alzheimer's. There is great promise for this. Likely it is best to use turmeric as much as possible in cooking. If this is difficult, daily supplements can be found (doses of 500 mg daily have been recommended, however as with any supplement be sure to use a reputable brand known for quality and purity).

The downside? Too much turmeric can affect the liver, so it should be used with caution in those with liver issues or taking other medications metabolized by the liver. Turmeric may also cause thinning of the blood and interfere with other medicines that cause bleeding. Do confer with your doctor if you have these issues.

A discussion of vitamins for memory and cognition would not be complete without mention of omega-3s. Their role in attention was previously discussed. They are felt to have anti-inflammatory effects, which may prevent or minimize cognitive decline. Some studies suggest a benefit to these "good fats" and some show no association with cognitive decline. It is our belief that omega-3s are generally good for you, but they are best found via natural food sources. If you feel the need to take a supplement, be cautious to find one that does not have high levels of mercury.

Caffeine for Memory, Too?

We know caffeine helps memory in the short term (not short-term memory), meaning taking it before learning new information seems to help with some retention of that info. Perhaps this is in part due to its help with attention that we discussed previously. What we don't know for sure is whether caffeine helps preserve memory over a lifetime. Some have theorized that caffeine has a role in preventing dementia. So, perhaps that cup of coffee is worth having.

One set of vitamins that has been suggested to have a negative effect on memory is heavy metals. Metals such as aluminum, copper, and zinc have been called into question regarding their role in causing Alzheimer's disease. Data has been conflicting, and this association has been challenged. However, it is our belief that one should avoid excessive supplemental doses of these metals. Iron deposition in the brain may play a role in Alzheimer's, but it is unclear if it is related to excess blood levels of iron or to some sort of defect that causes the iron to build up in unhealthy ways. There does not seem to be an obvious correlation between blood levels of iron (what we often seek to build up with iron supplements) and Alzheimer's. Therefore, it is our belief that taking reasonable doses of supplemental iron, when needed, is prudent.

Memory concerns are widespread and valid. It is our hope that thoughtful and judicious use of the right vitamins and supplements may help some of us preserve our memory as long as possible. No doubt maximizing our ability to attend to important things also plays an important role in our ability to live long and fulfilled lives.

CHAPTER 16
BLOOD PRESSURE

IN WRITING THIS BOOK, we felt a section on preventive health would not be complete without including our take on blood pressure. High blood pressure is such a common problem among adults that we could not leave it out. That being said, unlike some of the other topics we address, it is not a condition that is as readily treatable with vitamins or supplements. However, there are some instances where vitamins can act as part of a comprehensive regimen to lower blood pressure. There is a wealth of information out there on this topic, but we believe our perspective—after years of practical experiences treating people's blood pressures as a comprehensive part of their health and well-being—can be useful.

Blood Pressure 101

High blood pressure, or hypertension, is one of our greatest health problems. In fact, almost 30 percent of U.S. adults suffer from this condition. Perhaps "suffer" is a bit of a misnomer, since as with high cholesterol or early diabetes, this condition often causes little or no symptoms. In its earlier stages, high blood pressure often doesn't materialize as discomfort; people still feel well and have no complaints. It is only at more advanced stages that people may feel symptoms such as headaches, blurred vision, or chest pains.

The deceiving thing about high blood pressure is that you may not know it is present, but it can all the while be causing insidious damage. Its effects on the heart, brain, kidneys, eyes, and other vital bodily systems can be irreversible if left untreated. High blood pressure is one of the major contributing factors to heart attack, congestive heart failure, stroke, and kidney failure.

What causes hypertension? The vast majority of cases are what we term as "primary hypertension," which means a combination of genetic makeup and lifestyle factors cause blood vessels to constrict and raise the pressure. There are much rarer "secondary causes" of high blood pressure that have to do with hormonal imbalances, blood flow to the kidneys, or congenital problems. These unusual conditions need to be ruled out by your doctor in extreme cases of hard-to-control blood pressure. These conditions are far less common than garden-variety hypertension.

So what's the best way to find and treat hypertension? Firstly, *know* about it. Have your blood pressure checked at least once a year (more frequently if it has been running high). This can be done in a doctor's office, pharmacy, or in the comfort of your own house with a variety of home-monitoring devices (make sure to check your device against a quality monitor in a doctor's office to ensure it is accurate). Goal blood pressure is 120/80 or lower. Hypertension is defined as blood pressure of 140/90. The in-between region, of 130–140/80–90 is considered "prehypertension." In other words, it is a red zone that could progress to full-on hypertension.

First Aid for Your Blood Pressure

Jackie, a thirty-six-year-old woman, comes in to the office with symptoms of a sinus infection. She has nasal congestion and a sore throat and has felt pressure in her ears for the last ten days. When she first arrives, she has a blood pressure reading of 150/94. Jackie reveals she feels terrible from her sinus infection and has taken a "cold and sinus" medication this morning. Her mother suffers from high blood pressure. Jackie has not had an issue that she is aware of. She has three kids, her youngest being two. With each pregnancy she gained a significant amount of weight and did not entirely lose it. Currently she is twenty-five pounds over her prepregnancy weight. She feels stressed and at times overwhelmed with caring for her three kids. She also admits she has neglected to exercise or take much care of herself for this reason.

For Jackie, as for many people, simply knowing there is an issue can make a huge difference. In her case, this was the first time she was made aware that her blood pressure was significantly elevated. She was then motivated to take some actions to improve it.

———————◆———————

Once you are aware that you have high blood pressure, treatment options abound. Lifestyle modification is key. But depending on the level, medication may be advised by your physician. Though beyond the scope of this book, prescription medication options are in fact myriad (and ultimately effective once the right combination is found).

We would like to delve into some of the more natural ways one can tackle blood pressure. These techniques are useful at any stage of the game, but as with any chronic medical issue, the early bird gets the worm. It's always best to take action before you have significantly elevated blood pressure. If blood pressure is already well over normal, you should consult with your physician about the need for medication in addition to these strategies. Do realize that just because you start taking medication that does not mean that it is a lifelong commitment. With the right lifestyle changes (including diet, exercise, and proper nutrition) many people are able to eventually stop medication (under the supervision of a physician). Over the years we have stopped many people's blood pressure medications because they have gone well beyond their goal by making necessary lifestyle changes. Stopping medication is one of our favorite things to do (as long as it's done appropriately)!

Lifestyle Factors Proven to Lower Blood Pressure

Weight loss, even five to ten pounds, can make a big difference! This one really hit home for Jackie. She had slowly put on weight over the years and her blood pressure rise was somewhat of a wake-up call.

It is thought that increased abdominal girth puts pressure on the blood vessels to the kidneys and this in turn triggers the release of certain hormones that cause blood vessels to clamp down. Whatever the mechanism, losing weight is correlated with lowering blood pressure. This may in part be due to all of the associated lifestyle changes that typically accompany losing weight (like a better diet, less alcohol, and more exercise), but there is something intrinsic to having a lower weight that is helpful. And, as we know from other chapters, weight loss can also help many other chronic medical issues, such as cholesterol elevation and blood sugar. However, sometimes it is easier said than done.

In our practices we have seen very dramatic examples where people have shed extreme amounts of weight (a hundred pounds plus) and have been able to gradually and successfully stop all of the three blood pressure medications they had relied upon for years to control their blood pressure. Less medicine makes for a happy patient and doctor. A lot of weight loss certainly goes a long way, but even a modest drop can be significant and enough to avoid someone needing to start medication. Jackie's determination to lose weight was renewed upon hearing about her blood pressure.

Alcohol

Another factor to be considered in blood pressure is alcohol consumption. Sorry, folks—we know it seems like kicking back with a drink is just what you need for stress reduction, but sometimes it can backfire. Alcohol in significant quantities, typically at least two to three drinks in one sitting, is known to raise blood pressure. Limiting alcohol intake can be effective in helping to lower blood pressure. However, low doses of alcohol are also known to improve cardiac risk.

Sound complicated? We meet in the middle and advise drinking in moderation. It is not recommended one start drinking just for cardio protection, but if you do enjoy a drink, adhering to a moderate consumption is ideal. Typical recommendations include no more than an average of one drink per day for women or two for men up to age sixty-five. Over sixty-five, men are also advised to stick to one drink per day. So don't feel too guilty about enjoying a cocktail, just be sensible. Besides, who needs all those calories?

Exercise

Regular aerobic exercise is also key to lowering blood pressure. In addition to its help with weight loss, exercise itself has a good effect on blood pressure. While it raises blood pressure transiently for a few hours following activity (this is a normal response to exercise), the longer-term effect is to lower blood pressure. This may have to do with increasing the elasticity of the blood vessels and making them less stiff. It's also likely that certain hormones are released with exercise that ultimately dilate the blood vessels. Regardless of the mechanism, getting the heart rate up and the blood pumping is helpful here (as in most things health related!). (See the chapter on Exercise for more tips on ways to get started.)

An exercise goal of forty minutes *most* days of the week is advised. For blood pressure purposes, cardiovascular exercise is the priority, but some lighter weight training or resistance exercise can be mixed in. Good examples of cardio are vigorous walking, running, dancing, some forms of yoga, and swimming. Our patient Jackie realized she had let her own health habits lapse quite a bit in her quest to take care of everyone else. She was quick to say she could at least get in a good walk with the baby in a stroller and maybe even attend an occasional exercise class with on-site babysitting.

Caffeine

Another lifestyle modification that can be helpful with lowering blood pressure is limiting caffeine. It is clear that starting to take in quantities of caffeine when you did not previously shows a rise in blood pressure. However, for most people who take in a reasonable amount chronically (under 300 mg daily) there is only a slight increase in blood pressure. Therefore, we suggest no more than two caffeinated items per day (with a daily goal of no more than 300 mg). This does not mean two Starbucks venti double-shot drinks. This means two *normal* cups of coffee. We also advise avoiding any caffeine-containing "energy" products since they often provide large doses that can cause significant and potentially very harmful rises in blood pressure and heart rate. It is amazing how many people we see these days consuming large quantities of "energy" products (which is usually synonymous with high-dose caffeine) and not realizing the downside. Be very cautious with these. Rather, get you energy the proper way (see our chapter on this).

Nicotine

A real no-brainer when it comes to blood pressure is to stop smoking. Of course, this is easier said than done. Not only does smoking count as an additional risk factor for heart disease, stroke, and the other complications of high blood pressure, but it in itself raises blood pressure. It does so by causing the heart to pump harder and the blood vessels to clamp down. Stopping this nasty habit is the best thing you can do for your health hands down. It is never too late to start reaping the benefits. Cardiovascular risk returns to that of a nonsmoker just two years after quitting. It is well-worth the effort to kick this addiction.

Stress

A discussion about blood pressure would not be complete without mention of stress reduction. We all know that life these days is stressful by nature. However, one can still take the time and effort to find productive ways of reducing stress. Whether it's via a brief moment to yourself in the morning while the rest of your house sleeps, a coffee with a friend, yoga, meditation, or a trip to the spa, taking a moment to "unplug," both literally and figuratively, can make all the difference. When we created our packaging for Vous Vitamin® Personalized Multivitamins™, we were deliberate to include in each shipment the following instructions:

When you take your Vous Vitamin®, we recommend you take a moment for yourself. Turn off the crazy.

By taking this product you are already committing to help yourself and your health. Allow yourself a minute each day to reflect on that commitment. As you drink your water: think a positive thought about your life and about something for which you are grateful. Think about a future goal. Take a cleansing breath, and forge ahead!

We believe that everyone can benefit from this advice. Just a brief moment to retreat from the hustle and bustle of life can recharge you for the rest of the day. Doing so may be beneficial for your blood pressure.

Our patient Jackie really took all of this to heart. Once she recovered from her sinus infection, she started implementing some suggestions about how to take time for herself to recharge, focus on her own diet and health, and build in some structured exercise.

Medication

Before we delve into nutrition's role in blood pressure via both diet and vitamin supplements, we would like to touch on one of the less-talked-about but most common causes for high blood pressure we see in our practices: over-the-counter medicines. Many people chronically take common over-the-counter pain relievers or cold and allergy medications that can contribute significantly to raising blood pressure. Medications called nonsteroidal anti-inflammatory agents, or NSAIDS, such as ibuprofen or Advil®, Motrin®, Aleve®, and Midol®, can be toxic in many ways if taken excessively or with regularity even at low doses. They are useful medications for short-term injuries or ailments, and their anti-inflammatory effect is significant. However, one of their lesser-known potential side effects is a rise in blood pressure. (They can also cause ulcers, GI bleeding, and kidney problems, but those are stories for another day). Our best advice is to use them sparingly and only when needed. If blood pressure is running high, stopping them can often do the trick. Acetaminophen or Tylenol® does not tend to cause issues with blood pressure, and regular use in moderation is safer in this regard (but do follow the label's dosing instructions as too much of these are not good for your liver).

Likewise, some over-the-counter allergy or cold medicines, typically things labeled as "decongestant," "cold and sinus," or "D" formulations, are also notorious for causing or worsening high blood pressure. Many of these common preparations contain pseudoephedrine or phenylephrine. These medications work on nasal congestion by causing constriction of the blood vessels. It is therefore not surprising that one side effect can be systemic constriction of blood vessels, which—you got it—raises blood pressure. We recommend taking them only on rare occasion and for short durations of time. Many over-the-counter allergy preparations contain both an antihistamine and a decongestant. If you can get by with just the antihistamine you will not run into this issue.

Our patient Jackie had taken an over-the-counter cold medication the day prior to her visit, which may have played a role in her elevated blood pressure. Sometimes these medications do unmask a tendency toward higher blood pressure. People with this tendency should avoid taking these medications.

Birth Control

One other common cause of blood pressure elevation that we have seen in our patients is the use of birth control pills. While widely used and generally safe and effective medication for both contraception and other hormonal issues, these can on rare occasion cause someone's blood pressure to rise. If you recently changed pills or started taking the pill, your blood pressure should be checked. If elevated, it is sometimes worth stopping the medicine for a period of time and switching to another drug to see if this helps. It is often hard to predict when this relatively rare side effect will occur, but it's certainly worth considering before adding another medicine to control blood pressure.

Diet

Dietary changes can go a long way for blood pressure reduction. Reducing sodium can be highly effective for some people. However, some people are more sensitive to salt than others. Some recent research called sodium restriction into question. They questioned whether low sodium intake actually had a positive effect on mortality. It is true that this issue is still not fully understood. However, many years of research does show that lowering sodium can improve blood pressure in many people. For this reason, we believe that people with blood pressure issues should be cognizant of their sodium intake.

One simple place to start is with avoiding processed foods. Most packaged foods, especially frozen foods and canned soups, are full of sodium. Another surprisingly high contributor to sodium intake is store-bought bread. Most brands contain 250–300 mg of sodium per slice. Deli meat is also a culprit. So watch out for that sandwich, chips, and a pickle! You could be getting a whole day's worth of sodium right there.

Sticking to a diet comprised of whole foods such as unprocessed fruits, vegetables, lean meats, nuts, and whole grains is a great way to avoid many of the culprit additives found in most processed foods. (See the Nutrition chapter for more information.)

Sodium

Minimizing added salt is also a good idea. Some believe that using kosher salt or sea salt is healthier. It truly is more "natural" with less additives; and in fact there is less sodium, ounce per ounce, than in traditional table salt. Cooks often prefer using these because it is harder to "oversalt" something if using these products. We are all for using these as your preferred salt at home. However, one fact to consider is that these salts do not contain iodine, while traditional "table salt" does. The wider adoption of using noniodized salt contributes to iodine deficiency, which then can lead to thyroid problems. Iodine is easily replaced in a good vitamin regimen; just beware of this issue as you adopt a lower-sodium diet.

A general goal if you have higher blood pressure is to stick to less than two grams daily of total sodium intake. The "DASH" (Dietary Approaches to Stop Hypertension) diet is a group of dietary suggestions that have been studied and proven to help with blood pressure reduction. The program is sensible in that it advises using fresh fruits and vegetables, whole grains, legumes, and other healthful natural foods to make up the bulk of your diet. By sticking to these guidelines, you are less likely to consume the processed foods that tend to be the biggest salt contributors.

Is too little salt a problem? Of course it is! If you've read this far, you should recognize that moderation is always the answer. People with too little salt in their diets or those who take in excessive amounts of water (which essentially dilutes out the salt in their blood stream) are at risk of major problems too. Low salt in the blood or "hyponatremia" can cause people to feel poorly and in extreme cases can cause swelling in the brain, seizure, or coma.

People with lower blood pressure *need* salt to keep their blood pressure at a reasonable level and not get dizzy or pass out. Likewise, people who exercise a lot or are in extreme heat and sweat a lot also need salt at certain times to replenish their losses. You've tasted sweat (salty stuff); you lose a ton of salt and other electrolytes, not just water, when you perspire. When we created the Vous Vitamin® Power Up Situational Supplement™ for use with exercise, we worked hard to incorporate the proper balance of electrolytes, including a small amount of sodium, because we know that many people make the mistake of drinking tons of water when they exercise and not replacing the vital electrolytes too. Sodium is one of them, in reasonable amounts.

Potassium

The other component of the DASH diet that occurs naturally when you follow this type of regimen is an increase in dietary potassium. Following a diet high in fruits and vegetables tends to raise potassium intake since foods like bananas, citrus, potatoes, peanuts, tomatoes, fish, and whole grains contain significant amounts of potassium. The good news is that keeping a diet like DASH essentially kills two birds with one stone—lowering sodium intake while raising potassium intake. This winning combination can be just the recipe you need for keeping your blood pressure down.

Giving potassium in the form of a daily supplement is not recommended unless one has been shown to have a low serum potassium (a common situation for people who take diuretics or "water pills"). In part it is not advised to take too much supplemental potassium, because those who have imperfect kidney function can have trouble metabolizing the potassium. Also, their potassium can become dangerously high, causing heart arrhythmias. If one gets potassium from natural sources, one is less likely to have any problems (unless you have advanced kidney failure).

Magnesium

We consider magnesium to be one of the most miraculous vitamins. You have heard us wax poetic about it in previous chapters, no doubt. It is then probably not surprising that it can play a helpful role in blood pressure regulation. Some studies have shown a reduction of several points in average blood pressure among those who take a magnesium supplement. The exact mechanism for this is not fully understood. However, it is also known that magnesium is integral to keeping potassium levels adequate. Thus it may have multiple contributions to cardiovascular health. As with potassium, magnesium should be used with caution in those who have kidney problems. For most people it can be a good part of a heart-healthy regimen.

Vitamin C

Vitamin C is also involved in the complex equation of blood pressure reduction. It appears to be helpful in lowering systolic blood pressure when taken in addition to typical blood pressure medications. On its own, it has not been shown to be quite as helpful, but it may help in limited amounts. More research is needed to understand vitamin C's contribution. It may be one reason why the DASH diet is particularly helpful, since it includes many vitamin C–rich foods.

Calcium

Another element that may play a role in blood pressure is calcium. Studies, however, have shown conflicting results. It is possible that overdosing on calcium supplements can interfere with certain medications used to lower blood pressure (such as calcium channel blockers and certain diuretics). It is unclear whether they can be of any benefit in actually lowering blood pressure. We know they play a role in helping with bone density (see that chapter for more detail), but blood pressure may be another reason to take only the lowest needed dose of calcium via supplement.

———————◆———————

Clearly there are many steps one can take to help their blood pressure with or without the aid of traditional medications. Whether you just want to be healthy and keep your blood pressure where it should be, or you already have high blood pressure, many of the strategies we have discussed can be employed to help get your blood pressure where it should be. If you take medication for blood pressure or need to, using these techniques may help minimize the amount of medications you need to get your blood pressure to goal. If you put into action the strategies we have discussed, you will be working to optimize your cardiovascular health.

Our patient Jackie followed up two months after her visit for the sinus infection. Her blood pressure was back in the normal range at 136/86. Ultimately, her blood pressure goal is a bit lower, but at this point she has made significant improvements through implementing some strategies involving diet, exercise, and a thoughtful vitamin regimen. We are hopeful that going forward she will continue on the path to better health and lower blood pressure.

CHAPTER 17
CHOLESTEROL

CHOLESTEROL GETS A BAD RAP. Most people cower when they hear the word—perhaps because they envision their grandparents long ago, eating strange, orange-colored margarine products in the name of "treating high cholesterol." Whatever individual images it conjures for us, this substance has been near the top of the list of things in our bodies we hope to "control" for as long as we can remember.

Cholesterol itself hasn't changed very much; it is still contributing to some of the negative conditions in our bodies, while also doing its job in many positive ways. The way we think of it, however, has changed quite a bit in the last few decades and is still evolving. In short, high cholesterol is not just your grandmother's medical problem anymore.

There are a few hard and well-proven facts, and some unproven nuances, to the cholesterol picture. For example, we know that reducing low-density lipoproteins (LDL), or "bad" cholesterol, is shown to reduce heart disease and mortality in those with risk factors for heart disease. On the flip side, we have not proven that raising levels of high-density lipoproteins (HDL), or "good" cholesterol is also helpful. We do know that not having enough HDL is a risk factor for heart disease, and common sense tells us that raising this level *should* help, but the data to prove that do not yet exist.

So, what is cholesterol, and what does it do for us? We all need cholesterol. It is an essential component of our cell membranes. Healthy cells need healthy membranes to keep the good stuff in and the bad stuff out. Our brains also use quite a bit of cholesterol to keep our nerves firing smoothly.

What's Wrong with Having High "Bad" (LDL) Cholesterol?

High blood levels of the "wrong" kinds of cholesterol can also cause harm by building up on the walls of our arteries, and, for some people, ultimately forming into plaques. If these plaques accumulate, they can clog the arteries and lead to such things as heart attacks, strokes, or trouble with circulation to your limbs. Obviously, these are not good problems to have. But by knowing whether you have high LDL cholesterol early in life, you can take measures to lower it and thus prevent this buildup. The goal is to not get to the point that your arteries are blocked before you take action.

To determine what is bad versus good cholesterol, simple blood tests can measure it (best to take this test after a twelve-hour fast—no food and only water). The blood test usually breaks down the results into the following categories: HDL, LDL, total cholesterol, and triglycerides. Once upon a time we looked at just the total number. But in recent years we have come to understand that at least one of these components is good for us, so looking at the total number can be misleading.

What Does High "Good" Cholesterol (HDL) Mean?

The HDL or "high-density lipoprotein" is actually protective to our heart and circulatory systems. It seems to be the hero in the cholesterol world, perhaps by neutralizing some of the bad stuff. It also may help to thin the blood, preventing clots that can cause blockages in those already-narrow arteries. For these reasons, we consider elevated HDL levels over forty for men (lower expectations there) or over fifty for women to be a good thing. By some systems for assessing heart risk, having high HDL levels can neutralize other negative risk factors, such as high blood pressure or smoking (still not recommended). High levels of HDL seem to correlate with lower incidences of cardiac events but unfortunately are not a stand-alone guarantee for heart health. They must be taken in the context of the whole cardiac risk profile.

How Can We Raise Our HDL Cholesterol?

There is no doubt genetics play a role in the world of cholesterol. Some people just have lucky genes. Many of us have to fight a little harder to gain entry into the high-HDL club. How can we do this?

First, exercise! We can't sing its praises enough. Not only can exercise help lower the bad cholesterols (more on those to come), but regular aerobic exercise helps your body raise its HDL. How and why is complicated; suffice it to say that exercise seems to burn off the bad stuff, and this tips the balance toward the good stuff. The data are still out as to whether raising this number truly translates into better outcomes, but common sense dictates that more HDL is a good thing.

As with many things in life, there is also a "you are what you eat" component to raising HDL cholesterol. There are many good cholesterol foods, and these do not include your grandmother's orange/yellow tub of margarine. Foods in nature like fish (salmon in particular), avocados, nuts, and olives, all contain lots of good cholesterol. Therefore, eating those foods is one great way to help increase HDL levels. They are fattier foods by nature and can be high in calories, so moderation is the key. However, the fats they contain are the good ones.

Other food products that contain plant sterols such as Benecol® can be helpful in raising HDL. Ground flaxseeds or flaxseed oil also can be helpful. The seed must be crushed or ground; otherwise your GI tract does not absorb the good nutrients. We recommend Bob's Red Mill® ground flaxseeds. These can be purchased in your local grocery store and then added to just about anything (cereal, pancake batter, baked goods, yogurt, salads, etc.), and you will barely notice they are there. Flaxseed oil can be purchased in either liquid or capsule form.

Red wine may also play a role in raising HDL. This may be the best news you've read so far! However, don't think that this is a doctor's order to indulge in unrestricted red wine consumption. Moderation should be applied. The optimal recommendation for women is in fact one glass of red wine per day. Men may indulge in a second glass until they turn sixty-five, at which time the recommendation goes down to one drink daily.

Perhaps the most widely used product for raising HDL is fish oil or omega-3 fatty acids. These are supplements that come in capsule, liquid, or gummy forms and are rich in the nutrients used to raise HDL. They may also provide some anti-inflammatory effects and are touted by some for their help with arthritis, among other things. However, they should be taken with caution—ensure that the product is free of contaminants such as mercury (a heavy metal that can be found in fish and cause significant toxicity). A high-quality product is essential and the doses must be significant for an effect, totaling at least 1,000 mg daily of omega-3s. Many people find certain fish oil products leave a fishy aftertaste or cause an upset stomach. Sometimes these things can be avoided by freezing the pills. A number of people with whom we have spoken prefer gummy formulations, but these can be costly, high in calories, and often require taking many gummies to get a reasonable amount of omega-3s. At Vous Vitamin®, affordable, high-quality omega-3s are an important goal in our next wave of product development. You'll find out more about their role in relation to LDL cholesterol later in this chapter.

Are There Medications to Raise HDL Cholesterol?

This is a matter for you and your doctor to discuss. A few medications such as niacin or other cholesterol medications (statin drugs) can be helpful for raising HDL. Unfortunately, they are either poorly tolerated (as in the case of niacin) or they are more useful for other things, such as lowering LDL or bad cholesterol (as with statin drugs). HDL cholesterol is more of a lifestyle project than a quick medication fix.

What about LDL: The Not-So-Good Cholesterol?

Lowering LDL can be achieved in a variety of ways—firstly, by minimizing your intake of foods containing this type of fat; the biggest dietary culprits are red meat, fried foods, high fat cheeses, and other foods containing trans fats. For most people, cutting down on these foods will lower their circulating levels of LDL cholesterol.

There is some decent evidence that eating ten or more grams of soluble fiber a day can further help with reducing LDL. You may have seen the famous Cheerios™ campaign to this effect. Fiber of course can be found in a host of fruits and vegetables. One easy way to start the day off with a healthy dose is to eat a bowl (¾ cup) of oatmeal with a serving of fruit. This usually provides a nice boost in daily fiber intake, and it's a tasty, filling, protein-rich breakfast. Another means to lower LDL is via exercise (also mentioned earlier as a way to raise HDL—sense a theme here?). The effect of exercise is less direct on lowering LDL than it is on raising HDL. However, exercise promotes weight loss, and weight loss in itself contributes to LDL lowering. Therefore, it makes sense that more exercise is generally a great step in lowering the bad cholesterol, while it also raises the good.

If lifestyle is not enough to lower your LDL or bad cholesterol, what can be done? The current guidelines for when to treat cholesterol with medication are in evolution. Our thinking now is somewhat different than it once was. In the past, we looked at LDL numbers and had various targets based on these numbers. For example, if you were otherwise low risk (no smoking, high blood pressure, diabetes, or major family history), your goal LDL was to be under 160. If you had major risk factors, like a past heart attack or diabetes, your goal LDL was below 100 or closer to 70.

As with many things in medicine, you blink and there is a whole new way of doing things. The newer guidelines force us to use a website or fancy phone app to plug a bunch of variables (age, sex, race, total cholesterol, HDL, and a few more) into a cardiac risk calculator. If your risk of a cardiac event within the next ten years calculates to greater than 7.5 percent or you have known heart disease, diabetes, or an LDL over 190, you've just bought yourself a shiny new prescription for cholesterol medicine. It's slightly more complex than this, but for our purposes here this is the general idea. Cholesterol medication is thus reserved for those more at risk for heart disease or stroke, which does make sense.

The commonly used medications are very effective not only at lowering cholesterol numbers, but also at reducing the cardiovascular risks associated with high cholesterol. Statins or HMG-CoA reductase inhibitors (it's a mouthful, we know—we had to go to med school before we could commit that one to memory) are incredibly effective drugs. They lower circulation LDL levels via complicated chemical means. The bottom line is they work and *they work well*—so well that sometimes they cut your LDL numbers in half!

However, as with any medication, there is a potential for harm. A small (but significant) number of people who take these medications experience side effects. The most common symptom is muscle aches or cramps. These can occur at any time during treatment (sometimes after one has been taking the medication for months or years). They can be mild to severe, but typically not the latter, and usually resolve within a few days to weeks after you've stopped the offending medication. However, a very small percentage of people (approximately one in 20,000) will experience a more severe form of muscle breakdown called rhabdomyolysis. This can be a serious or even fatal condition if not treated, affecting the kidneys and other organs. Scary as it sounds, it is rare and can typically be avoided with careful monitoring of blood tests when taking these drugs. Most physicians check liver and muscle tests for people on cholesterol medicine at least a few months after starting medication and then several times per year thereafter.

How can muscle aches be avoided? There is some good evidence suggesting that taking a supplemental CoQ10 in doses between 50 and 100 mg daily in conjunction with statin therapy can help reduce muscle aches. This makes sense, since these drugs lower levels of this enzyme in your muscles. It has also been our experience in medical practice that patients who are deficient in magnesium or vitamin D (two deficiencies that are common offenders in causing muscle aches) are more prone to the negative side effects of statins. Therefore, we encourage our patients to take supplemental vitamin D (as many or most are deficient) and/or magnesium prior to starting a statin.

The good news about statins is there are many to choose from and each individual seems to respond differently to each drug. Therefore, the person who has trouble with one can often switch to another and find success. This process can take time and patience, but it is worth it if your LDL is dangerously high and you are at risk for heart disease. Believe it or not, in the near future they will be able to test your DNA and determine which drug may be best for you based on your genes! This is not yet widely available, but stay tuned.

When our patients are skeptical about taking statin drugs (they seem to have gotten a bad rap in the lay press over the years), we challenge them to find a cardiologist who is not taking them his- or herself. Hard to do. Most doctors "in the know" realize that these are incredibly useful drugs in the correct context. As with anything, there is a proper time and place.

So consider disregarding the late-night television commercials about the evils of cholesterol medicine and the online chats where people detail their woes with these drugs. It's always fun to entertain the idea that the drug companies have pulled the wool over our eyes and have been giving us poison for their own profit. But study after compelling study tells us otherwise. These drugs are safe if monitored correctly and highly effective in reducing heart attacks, strokes, and death in those who need them. Listen to your doctor on this one!

What about "Natural" Remedies for Cholesterol Lowering?

While doctors and patients alike would prefer to use non-medication options for most conditions, sometimes a reality check is in order. Unfortunately, not all that promises to lower cholesterol is safe. Here's what NOT to take for your cholesterol: red yeast rice. This "natural" product touted for its cholesterol-lowering properties is not a good idea. It does in fact lower cholesterol. However, as we mentioned with the above medications, everything has its potential side effects. The problem is, this "natural solution" has the same potential toxic effects as statins, as it is a "naturally derived" statin. However, due to its "natural sources"—or more likely lack of FDA oversight in its production—the variation of potency from batch to batch and quality assurances regarding potential contaminants and additives is highly variable.

Some batches of red yeast rice have been found to contain significant levels of toxins that can cause kidney damage, as well as chemicals found in prescription statins. Most people taking red yeast rice products are also not getting the proper monitoring with bloodwork as they would be on a prescription medication. Our best advice is to stay away! If you need to take something for cholesterol, take something that is a known FDA-regulated entity and under the proper medical supervision. In this case, the "natural" cachet is not necessarily better.

Another more "natural" prescription or nonprescription treatment option for cholesterol is niacin. This B vitamin was used for decades to treat high cholesterol, and it does help the numbers (lowering LDL, raising HDL, and lowering triglycerides). Sounds perfect, right? Not so much. First off, it typically has many side effects—intolerable flushing being the most common. Some people can handle this if they take it with aspirin. However, a few significant recent studies show that niacin may cause more harm than good. Large groups of people taking niacin had a higher mortality than those not taking it, which is a cause for concern. We do know it can cause serious toxicity in higher doses, causing liver problems, bleeding risk, and high blood sugars. It is probably best to avoid this one unless you have a very compelling reason (very high cholesterol and absolutely cannot tolerate other meds).

What about Omega-3 Products for Lowering LDL?

As mentioned in regard to HDL, fish oil and other omega-3 products can play a role in cholesterol improvements. However, these products, which contain important chemicals called DHA and EPA, are far more useful in raising HDL and lowering triglycerides (more on this soon) than in aiding in lowering LDL. In fact, high doses of fish oil can in fact raise LDL slightly. It remains unclear if this raise in total LDL is in fact a bad thing as it could be raising the good components of the bad LDL cholesterol. (It's confusing—we know. There's obviously a lot to this, and new research is coming out daily.) The bottom line is that fish oil should be used judiciously and not solely for the purpose of lowering LDL. In addition, many preparations of it contain vitamin E and other additives that can contribute to increased blood thinning. Therefore, taking too much fish oil can put you at risk for excessive bleeding.

What about Triglycerides?

We've discussed the good and the bad in the world of cholesterol, and now we bring you the ugly. Triglycerides are another type of cholesterol. They influence your total cholesterol value, and they also likely play a role in heart disease. Their role is still not as well-defined as those of HDL and LDL cholesterol. Triglycerides tend to be associated with high blood sugars and diabetes, but not always. Sometimes high triglycerides can be a first sign of another underlying medical problem, such as diabetes or hypothyroidism.

Some people have extremely high triglycerides (think eight to ten times the normal values) due to certain familial genetic conditions. In addition to conferring cardiac risk, extremely high triglycerides can put you at risk for a potentially lethal condition called pancreatitis (an inflammation of the pancreas). In these cases, triglycerides need to be treated promptly as a serious condition. For lesser elevations in triglycerides, the numbers can and should be addressed in a more stepwise approach.

The triglyceride value is very sensitive to what you have recently eaten as well as exercise habits. Thus, these numbers can often be improved via lifestyle. What does that involve? You guessed it! Diet, exercise, and weight loss—our staple activities for curing most of what ails you. The good news is it usually works really, really well for triglycerides. Losing a few pounds also can make a huge difference. Likewise cutting down on both high fats (especially saturated fats) and high-sugar or high-carb foods can dramatically reduce triglycerides in a short period of time. Notorious offenders include alcohol, fried foods, and, interestingly, certain forms of juicing. Juicing processes that remove fiber from the fruit tend to create a high sugar load without the fiber there to balance out the sugars as they digest. This causes massive amounts of sugars to be digested rapidly and quickly converted to triglycerides. Juicing is good to a point, but make sure the whole fruit is included so as not to lose this valuable fiber. We recommend talking to your doctor before juicing if you have a known triglyceride problem.

Some nonprescription options for reducing high triglycerides include omega-3s (discussed above for their use with HDL raising) as well as a prescription version of these (which is known to be high quality and pure). While niacin, as discussed previously, is effective at triglyceride lowering, its overall value and safety has been called into question. Few people tolerate it anyway, given its rather common side effect of severe flushing.

We do not tend to treat triglycerides with prescription medication unless they are at least double the normal range. The prescription options include the "fibrate" family. These drugs are not used nearly as much as the statins are used for LDL cholesterol. However, this may change as the relationship of high triglycerides to developing heart disease is more clearly understood. Fibrates are generally safe but are known to cause similar muscle and liver issues as the statins can. For this reason, similar caution and monitoring should be used. The incidence of these issues goes up several fold if the two types of drugs are used simultaneously (one for LDL lowering and the other for triglyceride lowering), so this should be done with extreme caution.

As with most cardiac risk factors, diet, exercise, and weight loss can carry you far and should be your first mode of defense against these risk factors.

So that's the skinny on fat and cholesterol. Get to work today on getting your lipid profile in the prescribed range; your heart and circulatory system will benefit immensely.

	HIGH RISK	COULD BE BETTER	IDEAL
Total Cholesterol	>240	201–239	<200
HDL ("good")	<40	40–50	>60(F) or >50(M)
LDL ("bad")	>190	101–159	<100 (70 is great)
Triglycerides	>500	150–300	<100

Cholesterol is an important and complicated matter. However, it can be optimized with a variety of lifestyle modifications. Genetics certainly contribute to how one's body metabolizes cholesterol, but diet and exercise can play a huge role in both raising the good and lowering the bad forms. Vitamins and supplements can be a great adjunct to addressing cholesterol but should not serve as a complete substitute for doctor-prescribed therapies when appropriate. Understanding your own cardiac risk factors so you can work to reduce them is the best way to get ahead of the game in protecting your heart.

CHAPTER 18

VITAMINS FOR BLOOD SUGAR AND DIABETES

WHILE WE HAVE TOUCHED on vitamins to help prevent various conditions, we debated the utility of including a chapter on vitamins for blood-sugar control and diabetes. Vitamins are not generally considered a typical part of the treatment or prevention of these issues, but it turns out there is some very compelling research that suggests vitamins can and should be part of the blood-sugar conversation. As an endocrinologist, Romy specializes in diabetes. She has found through research and clinical practice that vitamins can play a role in preventing diabetes and treating this condition as well as some of the many complications that can accompany high blood sugars.

In this chapter we will focus on type 2 diabetes, also known as adult-onset diabetes (Type 1 is beyond the scope of this discussion and unfortunately is not typically a preventable condition). Type 2 diabetes is characterized by the body's inability to process circulating blood sugar. The pancreas normally secretes insulin, a hormone that then helps metabolize sugar. In diabetes the pancreas starts to lose its ability to produce insulin and the cells in the body also become resistant to the effects of insulin. This does not happen overnight. Generally people start with fasting blood sugars that are mildly elevated (100 is the high end of normal), and this progresses over time to overt diabetes (fasting sugars over 140 or non-fasting sugars over 200). There is often a hereditary component to this, so people with a family history of adult-onset diabetes should be particularly vigilant about their blood-sugar numbers and preventive measures.

The good news is much of diabetes is preventable or at least controllable. There is a strong association between obesity and diabetes. Higher body weight seems to tax the pancreas and trigger elevated sugars. For this reason, all of the techniques we have discussed in regard to weight loss are likely to prove useful in diabetes prevention. Exercise is key to burning off the sugar. How to keep a diabetic diet is worthy of its own volume, but many of the principles we cover in our nutrition chapter are vital components of this (like minimizing simple carbs and balancing meals with protein and fats).

It is also important to understand that blood sugar issues have detrimental effects throughout the body. High blood sugars negatively affect the arteries, leading often to heart disease, eye problems (blindness is the extreme result), kidney problems, trouble fighting infections, and nerve pain (neuropathy). The main goal of treating blood sugars is to prevent all of these complications. Traditional diabetes medications (both pills and insulin) typically address the blood sugars alone, but we may turn to vitamins to also help with some of the potential complications.

First, we will discuss a few vitamins that are known to help reduce blood sugars and therefore slow the transformation of mild blood sugars to overt diabetes. Do keep in mind that these are rarely a complete solution to this very significant problem, but rather a piece of the puzzle of diabetes. All of the vitamins we mention should be one component of a comprehensive program including diet, exercise, and other medications your doctor may prescribe.

First off, there is some great data to suggest that vitamin D (one of our favorites) plays a role in blood sugar levels. One 2013 study showed that people with type 2 diabetes tended to have lower vitamin D levels. Those people with lower levels of D had worse control of blood sugar. The logical conclusion is that treating vitamin D deficiency should reduce rates of diabetes and improve glucose control in those who have the disease. Whether vitamin D deficiency is the cause of blood-sugar elevations or whether blood-sugar elevation somehow results in lower vitamin D levels remains unclear, but avoiding vitamin D deficiency, especially if you have blood-sugar issues or a family history of diabetes, makes great sense to us. (For many other reasons as well, vitamin D should be replaced. See chapters on Bone Health, Energy, Depression, Immunity, and more.)

Alpha lipoic acid (ALA) is both a water- and fat-soluble vitamin that has been used to treat elevated blood sugars. It reportedly somehow works to decrease insulin resistance, making the body more sensitive to whatever circulating insulin still exists. The benefits and dosing for this are still not clearly established, though a range of 600 mg to 1,800 mg daily has been used, with some reported success and little toxicity. While ALA may have modest effects on blood sugar, it is indicated as very helpful for diabetic neuropathy. The antioxidant effect of ALA seems to reduce the nerve inflammation responsible for this very painful and often debilitating condition. However, the most compelling data for ALA is with IV dosing. In our opinion, taking ALA orally may be worth a try, but it is by no means an absolute must-have in a vitamin regimen for diabetes.

Biotin (vitamin B7) has been shown to have some effect on lowering blood sugars. It is likely more effective when combined with chromium. Both of these vitamins play a role in energy and carbohydrate metabolism. This combination has also been used for treating diabetic neuropathy and pain, with fairly conclusive evidence in its favor. The doses studied are 600 mg chromium and 2 mg of biotin daily. Some sources recommend much higher doses of biotin (up to 10 mg daily), but we believe this amount is extreme and exceeds the U.S. recommended daily allowance (RDA) for biotin by a factor of 300.

A commonplace ingredient that can also be taken as a supplement is cinnamon. This spice has been shown to reduce fasting blood-sugar levels. While the evidence is compelling, how much is the right amount to consume or take in supplement form requires further research. There are also different types of cinnamon. The less expensive and more common Cassia type can cause liver damage in very high doses. Safer, but somewhat harder to come by, the Ceylon variety may be a better choice if using high doses. Since exact effective and safe doses of supplements are as yet unclear, it is our belief that consuming cinnamon via diet is probably the best approach. The Ceylon variety is preferable and can be added to a variety of foods daily for those with concerns about blood-sugar elevation. This can be a great addition to a comprehensive regimen to address blood sugars and try to prevent progression to overt diabetes.

One supplement that has a relationship to blood sugar is magnesium. This elemental electrolyte is often lost by the kidneys in those who have high blood sugars. For this reason many people who have diabetes or elevated sugars are deficient in magnesium and should replace it. For those who do not have overt diabetes, the question of whether supplementing magnesium can help keep blood sugars low remains unanswered. In one large 2003 study, people with higher serum magnesium levels were shown to have less of a chance of developing diabetes. Because most of us could use more magnesium for a number of reasons (see our Body Aches, Blood Pressure, and Migraine chapters), we do believe that this is generally a good, safe supplement to take in the proper doses (typically no more than 400 mg daily). Its potential risk is GI side effects (though many with IBS see improvement in their symptoms), and it should not be taken by people with known kidney failure.

A number of B vitamins have been suggested to be helpful for diabetes and some of its complications. Within the medical community, it is well-known that vitamin B12 plays a vital role in nerve function, and that B12 deficiency can cause numbness, tingling, and nerve pain. These are the very same symptoms seen with elevated blood sugars and what is termed diabetic neuropathy. Interestingly, people with diabetes are more likely to be deficient in B12. This seems to go along with the condition and can also be due to certain medications (metformin) used to treat blood sugars.

While diabetic neuropathy can exist even in someone who is not B12 deficient, it certainly makes sense for those with blood-sugar concerns to consider B12 supplements to correct the deficiency. They can have a blood level checked or can act with an eye toward prevention and take a low-dose B12 as part of a multivitamin. It has not been proven that correcting B12 levels actually prevents blood sugars from rising, but taking B12 in no way seems to raise blood sugar. It provides the additional benefit of potentially improving any signs or symptoms of diabetic neuropathy.

B6 is a vitamin that also plays a role in energy and nerve function. Some have recommended its use in moderate doses (100 mg daily) for diabetes or for diabetic neuropathy. However, the data for this is not overwhelmingly convincing. We do not believe B6 is likely to play a significant role in the treatment or prevention of diabetes and its complications.

Niacin, also a B vitamin, has been often used for its treatment of cholesterol problems (see the Cholesterol chapter for more information). It is known to lower triglycerides, raise good cholesterol, and lower bad cholesterol levels. Given that diabetics tend to have issues with high triglycerides and low HDLs, this is compelling. However, the problem lies in that niacin actually raises blood sugar. Therefore, diabetics must use it with extreme caution.

The omega-3 fatty acids, DEA and DHA, found in high concentrations in fish oil supplements, are similar in their ability to help lower triglycerides and raise HDL (good cholesterol). However, they too may raise blood sugars, though perhaps not to the same extent as niacin. Most people with high blood sugars tend to have high triglycerides and low HDLs as part of what is called metabolic syndrome. Therefore, fish oil would seem to make great sense in helping lower their cardiac risk. We believe there is still a role for fish oil and that people with blood-sugar issues should be monitored to see if the fish oil is causing significant rises in sugars (in our experience, its blood-sugar effects are minimal). Many will not be affected and can therefore continue the fish oil. Do note that excessive use of fish oil can also interfere with blood clotting, so most physicians recommend stopping fish-oil products a week prior to any surgical procedure to minimize potential bleeding complications.

Blood sugar and diabetes are significant concerns for so many of us. In fact, as of 2012, almost 10 percent of the U.S. population has full-blown diabetes. Another 25 percent of the population had elevated blood sugars or "prediabetes." These numbers are staggering and on the rise. This suggests than many of us should be actively working to improve our blood sugars. While diet and exercise are the cornerstones to diabetes prevention, vitamins too can be a part of the solution. In addition, people with known diabetes can make vitamins a part of their efforts to create a lifestyle and medication plan to optimize their sugars. Some of the more troublesome complications of diabetes, such as neuropathy, can also improve with the correct vitamin supplementation. As with any major health issue, there is no single solution for everyone; rather, each person should incorporate a variety of solutions based on his or her diet and unique health history.

PART FOUR:
BEYOND VITAMINS

CHAPTER 19
SCREENING TESTS

WE HAVE DISCUSSED THE ROLE OF VITAMINS in disease prevention at length; but as conscientious doctors, we would be remiss in discussing disease prevention if we did not explore the role of screening tests. Just as our patients over the years have expressed confusion about what vitamins to take, many also have heard conflicting advice about the importance and timing of certain tests. In this chapter we would like to weigh in on each of the most commonly recommended tests and when and for whom they are best done.

So much of what we do as physicians is about not just treating disease, but trying to prevent disease before it happens. Preventive medicine is both the practice of promoting healthy lifestyle choices and screening for potential risks so that we can halt diseases from progressing.

During each encounter with our patients, we try to impress upon them steps they can take to live healthier lives. Whether it's via a healthier diet, a consistent exercise program, or better sleep habits, the goal is always to be proactive, think to the future, and push people to take positive steps to minimize risk factors for developing conditions. One of the most effective ways we can avoid or effectively address certain diseases is through aggressive screening for them. Knowing whom, when, and how to screen is both an art and a science—and, as with everything in medicine, there is tremendous and often conflicting research about various screening tests, and when and how they should be used.

An Interesting Example of Screening Logic Gone Awry

We believe strongly in screening and early detection. However, science also tells us that screening protocols must be sensible and proven efficacious, otherwise they can in fact cause harm. For example, the old habit of screening chest X-rays to look for early evidence of lung cancer has been largely abandoned. Once standard, X-ray was later determined not to be a sensitive enough way to screen for lung cancer. Even though it can find many tumors before people have symptoms, using X-ray for screening has not been shown to be helpful in improving mortality from lung cancer. In other words, finding those cancers early actually still did not help people live longer. Logic, unfortunately, does not always translate into better outcomes.

However, more recently, we have started using computerized tomography (CT) of the chest in select populations with much more success. Recent studies show some benefit to screening with this more sophisticated technology, which finds cancers much earlier. The new challenge is then to balance the risk of screening with CT scan (radiation exposure) with the benefit of the information it provides. As it turns out, *low-dose* CT is a form of the test that uses less radiation and still gives good information.

The latest recommendations suggest annual screenings with low-dose CT scan for those aged fifty-five to seventy-four who are either current smokers or have quit smoking within the last fifteen years and have a "thirty-pack-year history." This means that they have smoked either one pack per day for thirty years or two packs per day for fifteen years, and so on. Lifelong nonsmokers need not be screened, though they can unfortunately still get lung cancer. They, however, are not likely enough to get it that the benefits of screening would outweigh the risks and cost of screening.

The lung cancer screening example is a useful one in that it shows us that screening has its downsides as well. It can be costly and anxiety provoking and may cause its own health problems (radiation may itself contribute to cancers in high doses). CT scans often find lung nodules that ultimately turn out to be noncancerous. They may need to be followed with more frequent scans or biopsied to determine if they are cancerous. This can be quite an ordeal, but it is likely worth it if you are an otherwise well person and you are able to find an early and treatable or curable cancer.

Of course, the moral of the story is that it's never too late or too early to quit smoking!

Mammography

It seems like these days we see pink ribbons everywhere. And while breast cancer awareness has come a long way, we are still surprised by how many women we see who are uneducated or perhaps confused about the proper things to do for breast cancer prevention. It seems like everyone has an excuse to blow off this most important of health issues and neglect their annual mammogram (recommended for all women over forty, and for some with a family history of breast cancer even younger). Some people state that it is not necessary because they do not have a genetic predisposition. *Au contraire*, friends—*all* women (and some men!) are at high risk for this disease (some more than others), since one out of eight of us will get it at some time in her life. Only 15 percent of breast cancer is familial. No woman with breasts is exempt, so pay attention!

Perhaps one of the best advances in cancer prevention in the last century is mammography. Still the gold standard for breast cancer screening, this relatively basic technology is very much the most useful way for the majority of women to look for early signs of cancer or precancerous lesions. Mammograms are basically X-rays of your breasts, taken from a number of angles (they do have some radiation exposure but it has not been shown to cause harm). Mammograms are most useful for finding small cancers before they spread. These are seen as "clusters of calcifications," which can be found to represent early-stage or in situ cancers. Abnormalities found on mammograms need to be further investigated with either more detailed imaging or biopsies.

Newer modalities such as magnetic resonance imaging (MRI) are useful in certain high-risk groups (talk to your doctor if you have a family history or personal history of breast cancer). Also worth mentioning are genetic screening tests for familial breast cancer, such as the BRCA gene. Commonly found in the Ashkenazi Jewish population, this gene is well-worth screening for with a blood test so that options for prevention of both breast and ovarian cancers can be explored.

Despite recent "controversy" about mammography, it is still our belief that most women, starting at age forty, should have annual mammograms. When to stop having them is largely determined by at what age one decides she would no longer take action to remedy an abnormality—i.e., once a woman is old enough or has enough other health issues that she would no longer consider biopsies, surgeries, or other treatments for cancer, it is time to stop early detection with mammography.

We have much more to learn about breast cancer and its many, many forms. It is possible that in the future we will go more by genetic markers than by X-ray-based technology for our prevention. However, we are far from that reality. Unfortunately, mammography is uncomfortable and anxiety provoking in that it does generate many "call backs" (to get better views) and biopsies that end up being normal, but it works. So, for the present time we're best off sticking with this relatively inexpensive, noninvasive test that we happen to know works to both find breast cancers early and reduce the mortality from them. This is a case where early detection does help!

Technology aside, a monthly breast self-exam is still also essential. It is in fact the means by which the majority of cancers are found. Get to know your breasts and what is your normal. The best time to do a breast self-exam is in the shower, approximately seven to ten days after the start of your period, if you get one. If not, set a phone reminder to do it a certain day of the month. By all means seek professional help when something feels like it is not normal or has changed.

Pap Testing

The bad news: This less-than-pleasant test is still essential for most adult women. The good news: Recent guidelines allow you to have it done less frequently than in the past. Papanicolaou testing (or Pap testing) was the first wildly successful screening and prevention program. Prior to its widespread use, women in the U.S. (and throughout the world) used to die of cervical cancer in the hundreds of thousands each year. As of 2015, about 3,000 women each year died from this disease in the United States. That is quite an improvement from what was once the leading cause of cancer death in this country. Many countries worldwide have not been as fortunate as we are to have instituted widespread Pap testing.

This simple, inexpensive test is not something most of us look forward to, but in the realm of preventive medicine it is nothing short of a modern-day miracle. Cells scraped from the cervix are placed in a solution and then viewed for changes suggestive of various stages of precancerous and cancerous lesions. If these abnormal cells are found early enough, simple office procedures can often prevent further progression of the disease.

Current recommendations are for women age twenty-one to twenty-nine to have Pap testing done every three years. Ideally, women ages thirty to sixty-five should have Pap and HPV testing ("co-testing") done every five years or, less desirably, Pap testing every three years. In the past, Pap testing was done without the addition of the specific HPV testing. (Human papillomavirus is the most common sexually transmitted disease in the U.S. While it often will go away on its own, it can cause genital warts and cancer in some.) Pap testing is not needed after age sixty-five unless a woman has a history of abnormal Pap testing. If a woman has had a hysterectomy with removal of the cervix as well, then Pap testing is no longer indicated.

There is one hitch to the reduced frequency of Pap testing now recommended: This does not necessarily mean fewer trips to the gyno. The Pap test is only part of your experience there. As part of a thorough gynecology visit, the practitioner also does a "bimanual" or pelvic exam where they feel your ovaries and other "lady parts" to check for any masses or other abnormalities. Don't skip this stuff! So continue to make an annual gynecology visit part of your good-health habits.

Bone Density

Perhaps the easiest screening test, a bone density test (DEXA) is a nuclear-based scan that involves lying on a table for a few minutes. It's really that simple. You don't even have to get undressed! This is how we assess risk for osteoporosis (see more on this in the Bone Health chapter).

Following bone density over a period of time is a useful tool in assessing risk for fragility fractures. Typically, a woman's first bone-density test should be done around the onset of menopause. It should be done sooner if you are higher risk for bone loss, such as if you have taken oral steroids long term, have taken excessive amounts of thyroid medication, or have had multiple unjustified fractures or other conditions that predispose you to bone loss (like celiac disease, hyperthyroidism, hyperparathyroidism, and IBD). Once a baseline is obtained, testing is typically done every two years thereafter.

Colonoscopy

Of course we've saved the best test for last! A colonoscopy is a much discussed, often feared, and possibly the grossest idea for a test ever. But guess what? It's actually not that bad. In case you are unfamiliar with the concept, this is the test where you spend one day eating no solid food. As if that's not bad enough, around 5 p.m. the day before the procedure you start drinking a "prep" solution, which is a nasty-tasting liquid that makes your bowels move like never before. It's sort of like the ultimate "cleanse." Suffice it to say you will be spending many hours in the bathroom. In the words of comedian Dave Barry, "And then, when you figure you must be totally empty, you have to drink *another* liter of MoviPrep®, at which point, as far as I can tell, your bowels travel into the future and start eliminating food that you have not even *eaten* yet." Sometimes the instructions tell you to stop drinking the foul drink once you're pooping clear liquid. You do actually get to that point. Sound like fun yet?

In the morning, you get to make your way to wherever you may be having the procedure done (with acute awareness of every bathroom in between there and your house). At that point, things take a turn for the better. You get a comfy bed, answer some standard pre-op questions, and take some good drugs to relax, and that's the end of your active participation in this procedure. You are given anesthesia and are essentially asleep for it, so the next thing you're aware of will likely be that the doctor talked to you after the procedure, but you have no recollection of what he or she said.

The good news is that we have convinced literally *thousands* of people to have this test done over the years, and *no one* has come back mad. You just get through it. The worst part may in fact be the whole no-eating-solid-food thing. You do tend to drop a few pounds, though this is not our recommended means to jump-start your weight-loss plan.

Why would anyone in the world advise this or actually go through all of this? Actually, a colonoscopy is a great screening test. It is in fact the gold standard screening for colon cancer. The other more antiquated modalities are beyond the scope of this book and are largely falling out of favor. A colonoscopy is an amazing test because it not only looks for polyps, the precursors for colon cancer, but it also removes them so they cannot become cancerous. The other screening tests—hemoccult (checking for blood in stool) and "virtual" colonoscopies (using CT or MRI to visually inspect the colon)—still require a colonoscopy if anything abnormal is found to actually deal with the problem (like burning off abnormal, potentially precancerous growths).

Who is lucky enough to have a colonoscopy? For starters, *everyone* age fifty and up. That means if you are fifty-five and have not yet had one, you are five years late and better get crackin'. If your colonoscopy shows no polyps, you can usually wait a full ten years to have another one (unless you have a significant family history or other risk factors). If you have polyps, you may be advised to have a follow-up test sooner. We often start screening colonoscopies before fifty for people with family histories of colon cancer in a first-degree relative. Generally, it is advised to start screening ten years prior to the age that person was first diagnosed. This is based on the concept that colon polyps are thought to take ten years to progress into cancer. Colonoscopies are also done at any age for evaluation of certain symptoms such as blood in the stool, abdominal pain, or a significant change in bowel habits.

Bloodwork and More

Needless to say, blood testing is a complicated issue, and there are many possible tests that can and should be done at different times in life. There is a multitude of guidelines out there about frequency of blood testing. It is our general belief that most adults should have annual fasting bloodwork for a few basic things: a complete blood count, basic chemistry profile, and cholesterol and thyroid screening. While checking for various vitamin levels such as vitamin D or B12 can be useful, they are not always needed in everyone. These should be done in conjunction with your doctor for specific reasons.

Annual electrocardiogram (EKG) testing (to look at your heart) is no longer the standard of care. Rather, EKG should be done for certain people in certain circumstances. That being said, it is our belief that everyone should have a baseline EKG for reference, and certain people should have them on a more regular basis (i.e., those with high blood pressure).

Pulmonary function testing (also called spirometry) or a "breathing test" should be done at least every several years for those with a significant smoking history to screen for emphysema.

———— • ————

All in all, there are some regular screening tests that just about everyone should have done. However, as with most things, there is a time and a place for everything. Guidelines and standards need to be taken into account, as do individual circumstances. When doing any test, it should always be considered whether or not the results would change what you do. If it would not, then it is generally not worth doing the test. For example, if you do a mammogram on a ninety-year-old woman, it is best to do the test only if you would follow through with some kind of intervention or treatment if an abnormality were found.

Proper screening is an essential part of good health. We believe that many problems can be avoided if the right testing is done and early intervention is applied when appropriate. Knowing when you should be tested and how often is an important part of maintaining your optimal health. Not everyone requires the same screenings. Individual and family history should be factored in to be certain that screening is done judiciously and appropriately.

While diet, exercise, and an appropriate vitamin regimen can go a long way toward bettering your health, screening tests should not be overlooked. They provide essential knowledge that can then inform your decisions about other measures to take toward improving your health.

CHAPTER 20
WEIGHT LOSS

PATIENTS ASK US ALL THE TIME how they can lose weight. Sometimes they are interested for vanity's sake, sometimes for their health's sake, and sometimes we initiate the conversation as we encourage them toward better health. As we discuss in other chapters, losing weight for those who are over their ideal body weight can be helpful for everything from treating fatigue to lowering cholesterol, lowering blood pressure, and more. The question is how to do it in an effective and lasting way. As with many other issues, the answer is not exactly the same for everyone, but some of the guiding principles can be applied to just about every individual.

One of our most popular blog posts on our Vous Vitamin® site is called "Click Here for Immediate 20-Pound Weight Loss." If you wish it to be that easy to lose weight, you are not alone. Everybody seems to hope we are going to offer up that magic pill, or that quick-and-easy solution that will make the pounds melt away. Sorry. No such luck. Losing weight is a process that requires effort.

There have in fact been hundreds, if not thousands, of books written on the topic. In medical school we were taught that if there is a problem that has twenty different types of surgery used to fix it, it is likely none of these procedures work very well. If someone needs an appendectomy, there is basically one operation to choose from because it works well every time. Not so much luck in the weight-loss game. Seems like everyone under the sun has a different "solution." If the med school theory holds true, that means none of these options actually work well.

The reality is that there is one simple solution: lifestyle, lifestyle, lifestyle. Finding how to create a lifestyle that works for you is different for everyone, and identifying ways to make positive changes in this regard can be time-consuming and requires a great deal of effort, but the good part is that lifestyle strategies do cause long-lasting weight loss if the right approach is taken. The challenge comes in learning for each individual what can be effective lifestyle changes, including your nutritional needs (both via food and vitamins) and exercise changes. Finding the winning combination is guaranteed to pay off—as long as you stick with it. And truthfully, it does not take expensive programs, coaches, or pills to lose a moderate amount of weight and keep it off.

However, sometimes more drastic approaches are effective in the right population. Surgical procedures have a role for the morbidly obese—those with body mass indexes (BMI) over 30—who have failed using other methods. Procedures such as bariatric surgery can help with massive weight loss but are fraught with potential difficulties, including surgical complications, resultant vitamin deficiencies (from the GI tract's lack of ability to absorb), and, perhaps most significantly, failure to sustain lasting effects in some. People who are obese because of underlying eating disorders and compulsive eating will not necessarily be "cured" with surgery. Thus, careful psychological screening is essential to help choose proper candidates for surgery. Additionally, those with diabetes will not necessarily be cured either. Rather, they may achieve better control of their sugars if they can establish better eating habits and implement diet and exercise to lower their weight. A discussion of these procedures is beyond the scope of this book. Here we will focus on those attempting more moderate weight loss (a hundred pounds or less).

There are many medications on the market today with the indication for weight loss. Some are used "off label" for this purpose, meaning they are not FDA approved for this (but are for some other use) but doctors choose to prescribe them. Examples of these include topiramate (a medication used commonly for migraine prevention) and metformin (used for blood sugar). Others are specifically designed and used for weight loss. They tend to be stimulant-type medications, but there are a number of other newer drugs out there.

We do not particularly endorse the use of any medication just for weight loss. The reasons for this are many. Firstly, some are toxic. As we learned from the fen-phen fiasco of the '90s (involving the drugs fenfluramine and phentermine), and then Meridia® after that (also taken off the market for concerns about toxicity), harm can be done. We know that any medication can always have the potential to be toxic, but in the case of weight-loss medications, we find that the return is rarely worth the risk.

Many of the available drugs do produce modest effects. The problem is that these effects are temporary. In our many years of practice, we have seen hundreds of people take medicines to get that jump-start on the weight loss of which they dream. The problem is, the medicine acts as a crutch. It reduces appetite and some pounds come off. However, it does not teach new habits. The vast majority of people who intend to use medication as a jump-start to their diet seem to use it for a period of time with some success. However, they ultimately need to stop medication (sometimes because it no longer seems to have an effect). When they do, they invariably gain back the weight. This is most often due to the fact that while on the medication they were able to suppress their appetite enough to eat a limited and unsatisfying diet. Once the medication is gone, the appeal of keeping this diet is gone and the whole thing goes out the window.

Newer drugs for weight loss include Belviq®, a serotonin agonist. This drug almost resembles an antidepressant in its mechanism but seems to work to some extent for losing weight. Unfortunately, it has the potential for causing heart problems, and only certain physicians with a special license may prescribe it. This is a bit suspicious in our book. Another drug newer to the weight-loss scene is Victoza®, an injectable drug typically used for diabetes. It can aid in weight loss, but it can also cause nausea and some ill effects on the pancreas. These drugs are not a long-term solution. They are indicated for extreme cases and are also costly for patients, even when "covered" by insurance.

Medication aside, there are many simple things that one can do to help the weight-loss process.

First and foremost, make sure your nutritional needs are met properly even if you have been overeating. Just because you have been eating enough calories does not mean your body has received the proper mix of nutrients. In fact, the lack of a proper mix of nutrients may be the reason some of us overeat. We are never satisfied, so we keep eating—but our body is still not optimized.

Therefore, before you embark on a sensible weight-loss program, consider a vitamin regimen that is tailored to your specific needs. If you take the proper nutrients, you may find you crave high-calorie foods less and begin to eat in a more sensible way. Strike the right nutritional balance so that your body can respond more effectively to your attempts to eat smarter.

Additionally, supplementing your diet with nutrients can help restore energy—the lack of which also may be fueling bad habits (see the Energy chapter for more on this). When you feel fatigued, rundown, and tired (which you may feel because you are deficient in things like iron, magnesium, or vitamin D), you are much less inspired to be active and exercise to your maximum capacity. Rather, you are inclined to be sedentary and to feed that lack of energy with quick, high-calorie fixes.

If you correct these deficiencies, you can gradually regain the motivation and energy to exercise effectively. This too will allow you to establish a healthy exercise routine that will, in turn, promote weight loss.

A quick fix this is not. A vitamin or supplement will not cause you to shed pounds and fit into those skinny jeans again. Rather, taking the appropriate vitamins and supplements can help lead to a more balanced nutritional level, which, in turn, can be part of a comprehensive lifestyle remake to get you on a more healthful path. Yes, it will take time and effort, but your body will respond to your efforts to eat a more balanced diet. You also will find exercise to be an instrumental part of this journey and a boost to your mental and physical health.

What vitamins you need are of course variable and based on many factors. At Vous Vitamin®, our entire basis for the Personalized Multivitamin™ was the concept that we all have different needs. Our diets, lifestyles, and health histories vary greatly. For this reason, the amounts of vitamins we each should take is different. We created a survey that took many of these factors into account so that we could give each customer the formulation we felt fit their individual needs. (See our Vitamin Glossary for specifics on the most-common vitamin deficiencies we see and in whom.)

Many of our customers have told us that just by having their vitamin needs met, they feel that their general hunger level has decreased. It is as though a certain thirst was quenched. This has fueled weight loss just as much as the ability to exercise more regularly when they have stopped feeling so fatigued.

Those who harness their desires to lose weight and use it to really examine their eating habits and make positive changes go even further. Exact dietary recommendations are beyond the scope of this book, but suffice it to say any basic nutritional plan that requires you to be mindful of both food composition and portion control can be used to guide your routines.

There has been much controversy about different types of diets. Fat-free, carb-free, gluten-free, diary-free, vegan, and the list goes on . . . Perhaps, again, we come to that concept of too many different ways to do it probably means none of them work. Or perhaps they all work, just each for different people. We know one man who lost massive amounts of weight on a low-salt diet. Physiologically this does not make sense. Just avoiding salt should not cause weight loss. However, we conclude that the habits he formed in order to avoid salt were so healthful and different from his previous diet that he did in fact lose weight with this diet. He avoided all packaged or processed foods. *Voila!* For him, salt avoidance triggered a seismic change in his diet (that he could maintain), and this was and continues to be his key to a healthy weight.

Studies have shown that simply keeping track of what you eat, via some kind of log (old school with a pen and paper or via various phone apps), triggers weight loss. It's true. Just writing down everything that goes into your mouth actually makes you lose weight. Perhaps it makes you consider carefully what you eat. Or perhaps it makes you slow down a bit and contemplate your eating a bit more, so you don't shovel in useless calories.

We are huge advocates of weight-loss programs that help participants monitor food consumption. Most do not provide any miraculous secrets but set up a framework that holds people accountable for what they eat. This can be done both by keeping track of food intake and having some accountability either by sharing it in person to a coach or with a group, or via online or phone apps where you get feedback on your progress. This has so many great implications for people's success. Not only do they have to keep track of what they eat, but in the group model they also can support one another and learn from each other's failures and successes. The online programs provide immediate feedback, as well, and sometimes suggestions for ways to improve. We are big fans of Weight Watchers®, because it is inexpensive, easy to do (great for people who eat out often or travel), and, most importantly, it is a sustainable program. You can stay on some form of this plan for the rest of your life and not feel deprived. Other plans, which provide you with complete meals, can be effective but tend to lead to the same issues with maintenance that happens with medications. At some point you stop the plan and you no longer have the tools to keep the weight off.

One of Arielle's favorite patient weight-loss successes is a woman whom she took care of for several years. Nancy was in her late forties and about forty pounds overweight. She took cholesterol medication and had slowly needed to increase her dose to get good results. She had struggled with weight her whole life, trying various diets and cleanses. You name it, she had tried it. She had essentially given up, citing her mothering responsibilities and work schedule as sabotaging her efforts. After years of discussions about weight loss (and her lack of it), the time came when her fasting blood sugar started to rise. Arielle provided her with a slightly stern warning that if she did not lose some weight and take other measures to lower her sugar via diet and exercise, she would have to start medication for this condition as well. Nancy's mother had been diabetic, so the news was particularly disturbing.

Nancy disappeared for a while and did not follow up as she was told to in three or four months. About eight months later she did return for an office visit. Arielle truly did not recognize her because she had lost almost thirty pounds. She was like a new person, her face glowing and exuding self-confidence. What had she done? She had used a program where she was keeping a food diary and watching calories and portion control closely in conjunction with a regular exercise program. She changed her eating habits completely. She managed to lose the remaining ten pounds over the next six months and has in fact kept it off for the last ten years. Nancy says she doesn't even think twice about her "way of life" because it is just who she is now. She has since gotten off cholesterol medication all together and has had no further issues with blood sugar.

Over the years we have seen thousands of patients whom we have advised about means to lose weight. The ones who have succeeded for a sustained period of time are invariably the ones like Nancy. They have made a 360-degree change in their lifestyle and that has enabled them not just to "diet" but to live a healthy life. Some have used structured plans such as Weight Watchers® or South Beach®. Some have found other nutritional programs that work well for them. Many have used vitamins to help their efforts. The common thread for all seems to be the lack of a "magic bullet." Rather, it's a lifestyle that works for them forever.

The Cleanse: Not-So-Clean Living

One popular phenomenon that might fall under the vitamin or supplement category is the cleanse. These consist of a range of different regimens intended to replace food for a period of time. There are many different versions out there, some as simple as a concoction made of water, lemon juice, and cayenne pepper; others made from a variety of fruit and vegetable smoothies; and others that are manufactured products such as shakes or beverages. All claim to "detoxify" and help give you a jump-start losing weight. No doubt, people tend to lose weight when consuming a liquid diet. However, the utility of these regimens should be called into question or at least kept in perspective when embarking on weight loss.

A liquid diet is by no means a sustainable way to live. Certainly one can get most of one's caloric and nutritional needs this way. But, let's face it, few of us would like to spend the rest of our lives drinking a concoction either bought in a bottle or whipped up in a blender no matter how "detoxified" we feel when we are done or how fresh it tastes. Therefore, these programs are a short-term way to lose a few pounds quickly. They are at best a jump-start to your new life-style. This is likely because your stomach does shrink after keeping a restricted diet. However, some people find they get hungry on them and then are ravenous for the few days following, which just defeats the purpose.

Some people find doing cleanses once or twice a month helpful. We, however, do not see them as a mainstay to a healthy weight-loss plan. No doubt, they can be a way to break your usual eating habits for a brief (one- to two-day) period of time and help you transition to a new lifestyle. However, we feel that most people do not use them as such. More people seem to use them as extreme measures to lose weight rapidly. As with the weight-loss pill concept, this is by no means a long-term solution or a sustainable habit. We believe your energy and willpower would be better invested in a well-thought-out, sensible plan for regular and ongoing eating.

There are many other herbal supplements touted for weight loss. In fact, a quick Google search for "supplements for weight loss" will yield no less than 54 million results. The possibilities may sound endless, but we again come back to our earlier-stated point: Millions of different substances are peddled for weight loss, and yet not one is really known to work in any sort of real or safe way.

A few products that may in fact work as they are supposed to include guar gum and Alli® (an over-the-counter version of the one prescription drug, orlistat). Both essentially block absorption of fat in the GI tract so your body does not take the fat and its calories in.

In theory, and sometimes in practice, people do in fact lose weight with these, but they can often bring on nasty GI side effects, such as abdominal pain, cramping, and sometimes loose stools and rectal leakage. Worth it? Probably not. They don't solve the lifestyle issue, though they may scare you into avoiding high-fat foods. As usual, you stop the drug and the old habits (and the weight) tend to come back.

Lately, garcinia cambogia has been all the rage. It is an exotic plant whose fruit's rind allegedly causes fat burning and decreased appetite. If you turn on the TV, you are likely to hear someone advertising its wondrous effects. Reality or good marketing? We suspect the latter. Evidence is conflicting and generally sparse in favor of this much-talked-about product. Even if it were to show some effect in the short term, as with other diet aids, it is unlikely to prove a sustainable long-term solution. In addition, it is known to have potential GI side effects, such as abdominal pain, diarrhea, and bloating.

Many of our patients come in asking about the Beta HCG diet (requiring injections of human chorionic gonadotropin). This craze, not unlike garcinia cambogia, sounds too good to be true—and is. It is a plan in which you severely limit your calorie intake (to fewer than 500 calories a day, which is, in our opinion, bordering on starvation). You simultaneously take some form of βHCG, which is a hormone that women's bodies naturally produce in pregnancy. The hormone is supposed to somehow reset your metabolism. It is absolutely true that starving yourself will lead to weight loss, whether you take a hormone or not. But there is no legitimate evidence that taking this drug (which is not FDA approved for any sort of over-the-counter use and is used only to help in some cases of infertility) will help you lose or maintain weight loss. We, in fact believe that you are much less likely to be successful at maintaining weight loss on this plan because of the extreme calorie deprivation. Starvation or near-starvation diets slow our bodies' metabolism, prioritizing only the bodies' essential processes. Once you revert to any sort of normal eating, your metabolism needs time to reboot and the food you consume will not be processed as efficiently. You are sure to gain back whatever weight you were able to lose. (Heard this story before?)

Ephedra is another herb touted for weight loss. It may in fact cause it. This is because it is a natural stimulant. It is a derivative of pseudoephedrine or ephedrine (used as decongestants). Therefore, it can cause all of the side effects of these things, such as palpitations, higher blood pressure, seizures, and agitation. Probably not worth the risk in our opinion. The FDA holds a similar opinion, since it has banned its use in supplements. Bitter orange is a similar substance, also banned from use.

The other latest fad in weight loss is green tea extract. It may in fact promote weight loss. This is likely due to its caffeine content. It may also help with weight loss because it contains a substance called catechins. There is more to be learned about this substance. These preliminary indications do not mean that taking huge amounts of green-tea extract is safe or useful. Rather, green tea may be your chosen source of caffeine. We advise it be used in its natural form (as tea), not in various products claiming to have super-high concentrations of its distilled contents. Many of these may contain other harmful additives. So, does caffeine really boost metabolism and, in turn, help weight loss?

A Word on Caffeine as It Pertains to Weight Loss and Health

People are constantly asking us about the effects of caffeine and whether they should kick the coffee habit once and for all. What we tell them might surprise you. Caffeine is not all bad—it does help increase metabolism and, in turn, this helps facilitate weight loss. Now, does this mean that ingesting large quantities of caffeine with hopes of trimming down is the way to go? Of course not. As with most things in life, too much of a good thing is not necessarily better.

One recent study showed that athletes who took in caffeine pre-exercise burned about 15 percent more calories for three hours post-exercise, compared to those who ingested a placebo. This suggests that the effects of caffeine, namely raising heart rate, do help burn calories, which, in theory, should assist in weight loss. Please understand that a conclusive study proving this has not yet been done; so these results have given rise to a theory rather than conclusive fact.

Can you take advantage of caffeine for weight loss? Well, the previously mentioned study suggests that about 300 mg of caffeine (which equates to a cup and half or so of coffee) before exercise actually has an effect on post-exercise metabolism. This may be one reason why people find morning workouts more beneficial. You, too, may consider moving your exercise routine to morning hours if you start your day with a cup of joe.

There has often been concern that caffeine causes dehydration. Simply put, it does and it doesn't. In the short term, it does. So, taking a big dose of caffeine such as one provided in an "energy drink" if it is not your typical fare, does lead to an immediate loss of bodily fluids (you might have noticed that you tend to pee a lot after ingesting caffeine). However, studies also have shown that people who ingest caffeine chronically in a routine manner develop a mechanism to adjust to the caffeine intake and lose less water. Therefore, a regular coffee or tea routine (in moderation) should not ultimately lead to dehydration. But, using large random doses of caffeine in the form of energy drinks or other energy boosting tablets/gels, etc. is not ideal, as it will likely affect your workout and subsequent hydration status negatively.

As we've said before, too much of a good thing is not always better. There are negative effects from too much caffeine. The side effects of excess caffeine can range in severity from annoying to lethal. Along with activating your central nervous system (thus the great effects on alertness and memory), it also activates your cardiovascular system. In turn this can cause your heart rate to go up, producing a sensation of palpitations (or in rare cases, it can bring on dangerous arrhythmias). Likewise, the stimulation can contribute to high blood pressure.

There have been several reported cases of seizures and death after ingesting large or unknown quantities of caffeine-containing energy products. This, of course, raises the concern that the megadoses available in these forms are not safe and should be avoided. There are added concerns when combining "energy" in the form of caffeine with alcohol. None of the energy products are FDA regulated, and it is of great concern that their contents are not rigorously tested. It is our belief that caffeine from naturally derived sources (coffee, tea, chocolate, and the like) is much less risky because it is harder to overdose.

The obvious side effect of too much caffeine is insomnia or interrupted sleep. What many do not realize is that this effect can be prolonged, lasting twelve hours or more after you ingest it. Another less-recognized issue with caffeine is the rebound headache. Caffeine has effects on blood vessels in the brain that can reverse migraines. Caffeine is, in fact, a common ingredient in over-the-counter migraine medications. It is useful for this purpose. However, the downside is that people who ingest caffeine regularly are prone to withdrawal headaches when they stop. The best way to address this is to moderate your intake and if needed wean down to a lesser amount that does not lead to this rebound effect.

For many of these reasons, a daily maximum of 400 mg of caffeine is advised. (See chart below for typical sources.) Do recognize that not all coffee is created equal. A Starbucks dark roast packs a greater punch than your typical Folgers (a Starbucks tall brewed coffee is reported to have about 260 mg per 12 oz., which far exceeds the typical cup of coffee listed below—this is in part due to the larger size of 12 oz. versus 8 oz.). Natural sources are likely a safer way to obtain caffeine than via high-dose energy drinks or supplements. When it comes to green tea, we suggest drinking actual green tea, rather than buying supplements that contain its extract. They are not well-regulated and may contain harmful additives (even if not listed on the ingredients) since there is little oversight in their manufacturing.

We also advise you stop caffeine intake after noon to minimize its impact on sleep at night. Its effects on sleep quality and duration can be subtle but take their toll. So enjoy that cup (or two) of java each morning before you work out, but otherwise limit your intake. Also, beware of the fact that many of today's specialty coffee drinks are paired with loads of sugar and fat. These can be a huge source of hidden calories that if left out can aid in a plan to lose weight.

Beyond all the lifestyle changes we continue to harp on, we have gleaned a few additional weight-loss tips, some from the scientific research, but many from talking to our patients who have had great successes over the years.

CAFFEINE CONTENT OF COMMON SOURCES:
Credit: WebMD

CAFFEINE SOURCES	APPROXIMATE CAFFEINE CONTENT (MG)
Coffee, regular (1 cup)	138
Espresso (¼ cup)	125
Cappuccino, regular (1 cup)	60
Latte, regular (1 cup)	60
Tea, brewed, hot (1 cup)	47
Nestea Iced Tea, Earl Grey (1 cup)	33
Cola soda, regular or diet (12 oz.)	42
Mountain Dew (12 oz.)	52
Chocolate, semisweet (1 oz.)	18
Chocolate milk (1 cup)	5
Cocoa powder (1 tablespoon)	12

A Few Tips on Healthful Eating

Planning, planning, and more planning. This appears to be most crucial in the early stages of a healthy eating plan. For those who work outside of the home, making lunches and snacks can be the best way to prepare for the week ahead so that one has access to "good choices" while at work and is not tempted to hit the vending machine, convenience store, or fast-food chains. Likewise, if you are at home much of the time, keeping your home free of too many temptations is helpful. Also, measuring out snacks in advance is useful (we have heard of people who literally measure out their snacks and meals at home as if they are packing them for the day, to avoid oversnacking or excessive portions). While this fastidious approach may seem like overkill, it is most useful early on when making changes. Portion control will eventually come more naturally as a habit once you have done it properly for a while, and you can likely relax a bit on the planning.

Sometimes a little bit of the "wrong food" trumps a lot of the better stuff. Years back, low-fat foods became all the rage. SnackWell's™ were thought to be the messiah of weight loss—low-fat cookies to replace the traditional Oreo® as a snack food. In the '90s, people thought SnackWell's™ might be the solution to the great American obesity epidemic, and people started consuming them in mass quantities. Not so helpful, right? Twenty SnackWell's™ still have as much fat and calories as a lesser amount of Oreos® and, let's face it, are far less satisfying. We are by no means suggesting an Oreo® diet. The point is you may be more satisfied by a smaller portion of the better-tasting food than by eating a massive quantity of the "healthier alternative" (some of which are questionable in the first place since they are equally high in carbs and sugar).

A more current example of not-so-healthy "health foods" are many of the gluten-free products. Some people find avoiding gluten is both a means to feeling better and losing weight. The reasons for this are manifold. However, do not fall into the trap of replacing lots of foods that would normally contain gluten with their gluten-free equivalent, like gluten-free cakes and cookies. Many (not all) of these products replace the gluten with very high-fat and high-calorie equivalents.

We believe avoiding gluten, if done right, can make for a healthful diet. It means avoiding the baked goods and high-carb foods that would normally contain gluten; and rather than buying many processed alternatives, stick to simple whole-food replacements. For example, skip the pasta and replace it with a small serving of brown rice or skip the starch all together. Instead of a bagel for breakfast, replace it with a healthful Greek yogurt and fruit. Make your afternoon snack some veggies and hummus instead of a granola bar. Replace the sandwich with a salad.

Gluten-free eating is not a magic guarantee for weight loss. However, some people find it a useful framework for adapting a healthier eating pattern. Remember, though, to think about the long game. If you feel that going completely gluten-free makes you feel deprived, it may not be for you. We have heard plenty of stories about people who have gone off the gluten-free deep end after months of feeling deprived, only to down a whole pizza or a pound of pasta. This defeats the purpose. There may be a healthy middle ground, such as a once-a-week splurge.

For example, we know of one woman who was put on a weight-loss program but allowed herself a pint of ice cream for dinner once a week. She was incredibly successful at losing and maintaining her weight loss for many years. We by no means endorse this as a healthy strategy. The point is that somehow that indulgence kept her on track the rest of the time. Find your controlled indulgence! We each have our vices and our weaknesses. Perhaps acknowledging that they exist and embracing them as part of an overall health plan is a more realistic and longer-lasting approach.

When planning, one must be prepared for potential weaknesses. The most typical time that people seem to stray are at events and parties, and of course this often occurs during the holiday season. One suggestion before these types of events is to "pre-eat." Some people starve themselves in anticipation of a big night out because they know they will be consuming so much. However, eating something slightly filling and healthy before going does not mean you cannot enjoy the offerings; rather it means you may have "taken the edge off." If you are not totally ravenous, you may be able to control what you put in your mouth more. So go only slightly hungry and choose wisely what is worth the indulgence. Also beware of the many calories in alcoholic beverages.

Speaking of beverages, a word on soda. There has been a lot of talk in the news regarding the role of "diet" sodas in weight loss or gain. There is no question that sugar sodas are full of calories and a huge contributor to our nation's struggle with obesity. While many people think sodas cause weight gain only if they are full of sugar, in reality even diet soda (no-calorie soda) has been shown to cause weight gain. One 2014 study in fact showed that artificial sweeteners are linked to a rise in blood sugar, which ultimately correlates with developing diabetes. For this reason and many others, we are not fans of soda.

A very crucial component to any weight-loss plan is exercise. Even a dramatic change in diet is best enhanced by a good exercise program. Most of the patients we have treated find that even a drastic reduction in calories eventually results in a plateau of weight loss without adding in a significant exercise program. We believe that improvements in diet and exercise done simultaneously and in a stepwise fashion are the most essential components to any sustained weight loss. The exercise habit seems to both mentally and physically solidify the dietary changes. Often people think that if they burn a certain number of calories exercising, they don't want to hastily "undo" all that work by eating poorly. Also, many people report that exercise actually reduces their appetites. This is not always true, however; the best way to avoid excessive hunger is to eat small, frequent protein-rich meals leading up to exercise to avoid the ravenous urge to overindulge after a workout is completed.

Not only does exercise burn extra calories when you are doing it, but it stimulates the release of a variety of hormones and chemicals that help keep your metabolism functioning optimally in between sessions. Muscle mass gets built up during regular exercise, and these muscles in turn burn more calories every day just to maintain them. (See more in the Exercise chapter for strategies to effectively incorporate exercise into your daily routine.)

Anyone with pounds to shed knows that weight loss is a challenge. There are many strategies one can employ to obtain effective and sustainable weight loss. Finding what works best for each person is essential. Because we believe weight loss is not about a "diet," but rather about a change in lifestyle, vitamins are a useful tool in this approach. Adapting to a healthier lifestyle can take many months to refine.

Weight loss that is done methodically and over time (no more than one to two pounds per week) is much more likely to be maintained in the long term. Remember, you did not gain it that quickly (though sometimes you feel like you did). Crash diets, cleanses, and stimulant medications have not been shown to have long-term success. They may cause quick shedding of pounds, but that often leads to weight gain once the quick fix is over. Slow and steady wins the race. Changing your life for the better is the surest way to change your weight once and for all.

CHAPTER 21
EXERCISE

WE TOUCH ON EXERCISE throughout the book in regard to its role in helping with many health issues: weight loss, cholesterol, high blood pressure, bone health, IBS, sleep, and more. While it is not directly related to taking vitamins, we would like to share our thoughts on exercise because of its importance in overall health.

Clearly exercise is an essential part of a healthy lifestyle for anyone. As with most things, exercise can take many different forms and people's preferences differ. But for everyone it should involve some sort of time dedicated to exerting oneself more than routine daily life requires.

This leads us to a common misconception. On the Vous Vitamin® questionnaire to obtain a Personalized Multivitamin™, we ask about exercise habits. The answer choices range from upward of an hour per day to "Does walking to the fridge count?" A tongue-in-cheek answer, this is unfortunately an assumption that many people make. When asked about exercise, we have heard dozens of patients over the years answer, "I'm on my feet all day; I'm very active." Does this count? The answer is yes and no.

While yes, an active daily life is certainly better than a sedentary one (studies have shown that those who sit for prolonged periods at a desk even when they have an hour of structured exercise are more at risk for health problems than those who do not sit all day), but we believe strongly that dedicated exercise time is essential. Not only is it a physical must to get your heart rate up for a sustained period of time, but mentally it helps to have some time to de-stress, focus on moving your body, and, in turn, centering your mind. Also, an active life alone does not usually supply enough calories burned to promote weight loss.

Guidelines suggest that ideally every person should be exercising at least forty minutes *most* days of the week. While it may sound like a lot of time to someone who is not in this routine, those of us who are habitual exercisers actually feel like our day is not complete when we do not have this time. The key then is, how do you get from being a couch potato to a habitual exerciser? As with anything else, creating new habits is time-consuming but can be done with slow, incremental change.

Sometimes looking at your existing day and schedule is a great place to start. When you look at your existing habits, you have a vantage point to figure out from where you can build. Gathering some initial data about what you are or are not doing also allows you to create some reasonable goals. It is unlikely that someone with a busy schedule with no built-in exercise time will suddenly incorporate ninety minutes every day into their routine. However, that person may find twenty-minute opportunities many days of the week or a larger block of time one or two days per week.

Tools such as pedometers or fancier phone apps and computer programs can be great for helping to track your steps, calories burned, etc. They are a great way to see how active you are in a day and look for ways to make improvements. Likewise, just as with diet trackers, the simple act of keeping a record seems to motivate many people to do the right thing. However, remember that number of steps are a great thing and we should all strive for as many as possible, but let us not forget that at least a portion of those steps should occur during a dedicated exercise time, not just being up and about in your home or workplace. Some of the more advanced models incorporate calories burned and heart rate, which can be useful tools.

The good news is you *do not* need an expensive gym membership and a two-hour-a-day commitment to fulfill an exercise requirement! Opportunities to exercise are all around you if you look for them. As with other aspects of help, sometimes taking a step back and reexamining your daily routine can shed a whole new light on ways to implement change.

A few possibilities include:

- Take the stairs whenever possible. We were taught in medical school that for the sake of time and health, we should always take the stairs. It is a great habit that has persisted. Unless you are in a skyscraper, taking the stairs a few flights can certainly be a quick health break.

- Park far away. It seems counterintuitive since we all crave "rock-star parking." But when it comes to health, we should all push ourselves to walk more.

- Instead of meeting a friend for coffee or a drink, suggest a power walk or a yoga class.

- Walk or bike to do errands or for your commute. Depending on where you live and work, many of us rely on cars or public transportation for routes that could easily be walked or biked. Take that extra minute to think about it and plan it, and you will not regret it.

- Start small. Going from nothing to ten or fifteen minutes a day is a huge improvement. We have seen too many people fail by being overly ambitious. Beginning a limited routine and gradually building on it is far preferable.

In addition to looking for opportunities around you, we also encourage you to find easy and inexpensive at-home exercises. Exercising in your residence can take on a range of forms. The most costly yet reliable in-home exercise plan is to employ a personal trainer, who either comes to you or works out with you at a facility. While this is a wonderful way to ensure you get exercise, it can be quite expensive; and for this reason people tend to limit the time they use this service, which can defeat the point. We believe quantity is more important than quality in this regard, so consider sharing the cost (and the workout) with a friend or getting a good routine you can do on your own in between sessions.

Since not everyone is inclined or able to afford the luxury of a personal trainer, home exercise can be started quickly and simply with something like *The New York Times'* "Scientific 7-Minute Workout." This is a well-thought-out series of twelve exercises that one can do for thirty seconds each, allowing for a ten-second break in between. It requires no equipment other than a chair and a wall. The whole routine totals seven minutes, and of course one can take the liberty to repeat it or lengthen the intervals. However, it is a pretty intense seven minutes and, even for those in decent shape, it can be a challenge. And really, who doesn't have seven minutes to spare? Excuses end here.

Another great free in-home exercise plan is yoga. There are instructional yoga videos galore online. You can choose from endless types of instruction, length of video, and difficulty level on YouTube or various dedicated websites (such as http://www.doyogawithme. com or http://www.myfreeyoga.com). Also, many cable networks have on-demand yoga or other exercise programs. Yoga is typically better for strengthening and flexibility than aerobic activity, though usually not as good a cardio workout.

One commonly recommended technique for lowering blood sugar is doing intense aerobic activity immediately after eating. Some people are hesitant to exercise immediately after eating, and that is largely due to the fact that intense activity such as running can cause GI upset or cramping for some. There is nothing inherently medically bad about lighter exercise after eating. Especially in people with high blood sugars or diabetes, exercising after eating makes great sense, as it helps to lower the blood sugar. Those who take medications for diabetes should be cautious to always check blood sugars before they exercise and not start if they have a sugar below 100 without having a snack first. Those with diabetes should also not exercise when their sugars are too high either, as this too can cause major problems. If you are diabetic, review guidelines with your doctor about when it is safe to exercise.

One convenient way to get a quick calorie burn without even leaving your own home is to use cans of food to do bicep curls—ideally, use larger cans, such as the 28 oz. size, and do several sets of thirty reps of bicep curls. There are numerous YouTube video series featuring a variety of exercise routines using soup cans. (If you choose to make this part of your morning routine, you can do your workout and then eat the equipment for lunch! Actually, watch the sodium in those cans—probably better to use them as weights.

Actual exercise equipment for the home can sometimes be found inexpensively online or secondhand, through garage sales or second-hand-equipment retailers. Of course, fancy equipment is by no means a must. We have had numerous patients report to us they get a great workout by literally running the stairs in their homes or doing various calisthenics.

Another thing to keep in mind when looking to get into an exercise habit is to find something you love. Of course this can be easier said than done. However, it is worth having an open mind to try different forms of exercise until you arrive at something that you inherently enjoy enough that it keeps you coming back for more. Arielle was not an avid exerciser earlier in life but took up running simply to get healthy. After a decade of running, she was bored and really dreaded it. She tried a variety of alternatives—yoga, Zumba™, weight training classes, Pilates, and more. Ultimately she discovered Cardio Tennis®, despite only having tried the standard version of the game briefly in childhood. Cardio Tennis® combines lots of running with hitting tennis balls and playing short competitive games. Classes are offered by some local park districts. It has become an addiction for Arielle! It is in part due to the fact that it is lively, with music playing and lots of people. Whatever the reason, it keeps her coming back for more and looking forward to it every time. This is the best kind of exercise: something that is genuinely fun.

Many people, particularly (but not only) men, seem to enjoy sports that involve chasing a ball. If this is what appeals to you, go find a way to do it. There are adult leagues for everything from soccer to basket-ball, floor hockey, volleyball, tennis, field hockey, softball, and more.

Most are low cost and easy to join. If this is what gets you excited to exercise, find a way to build it in.

Do not underestimate the role of socializing in exercise. The human connection can be a huge draw and sustainer for many of us when it comes to a routine. The simplicity of meeting a friend to walk or not letting down your team can be a huge draw in keeping you on track. A huge industry of competitive races has been built around this concept—people run everything from 5Ks to marathons largely to be a part of a big event with other people. Use this momentum to propel yourself into action!

As we mentioned previously, your ultimate goal should be at least thirty to forty minutes most days of the week of some kind of structured exercise. The question always comes up, "What is better, cardio exercise or weight training?" In our opinion, cardio should be the focus, with an eye toward whole-body weight-related activities (both weight-bearing and weight-training activities). This means you should focus your efforts on getting your heart rate up to targets (more on this shortly). How you get your heart rate up is less important, though some element of resistance on both upper and lower body is ideal. Almost any exercise regimen meets these criteria. We touch on weight bearing and its importance for osteoporosis prevention in the Bone Health chapter. Weight bearing is typically found as a part of most exercise activities, while weight training is usually more involved and attempts to actually build muscle mass using resistance and/or other equipment. Weight training, while more optional in our eyes, is desired by many for cosmetic reasons. But it's also helpful from an energy and metabolism standpoint, because muscle mass does raise your metabolic needs and therefore burns calories even when you are not actively exercising.

There has been debate about in which order to do your workout. Cardio first? Weight training first? A 2014 study shows little difference in outcome if doing cardio prior to weight training or vice versa. The research specifically looked at effect on muscle function. This reinforces our general belief that something is better than nothing and exact type or order is less relevant than doing a reasonable amount of exercise on a regular basis. Getting your heart rate up to target is important if you feel you are not getting benefits from your workout (i.e., struggling to lose weight or not feeling your stamina is improving).

The way to calculate your target (or maximum) heart rate is as follows:

85 percent of 220 minus your age

For example: if you are age forty, multiply $0.85 \times 180 = 153$

At age forty, a good workout target is to keep your heart rate close to 150 for the majority of your workout time. Heart rate can be easily measured by taking your pulse or via a multitude of available monitors.

Vitamins can play a crucial role in giving your body the tools it needs to optimally exercise. Your muscles need the correct electrolytes and nutrients to work their best. Vitamins essential to exercise include B vitamins, magnesium, potassium, and sodium chloride, among others. At Vous Vitamin®, we have met this need with our Power Up Situational Supplement™, created specifically to give you the electrolytes and vitamins that are helpful around the time of a workout. Taken with water, people find this tablet to help them perform and recover optimally. (See previous chapters on Body Aches and Energy for more specific vitamin suggestions.) Remember that hydration requires both water and electrolytes to be adequate.

Exercise is such a vital part of living a healthy life. It both prevents and treats so many health issues that no discussion of wellness would be complete without touching on exercise. While we each start in our own place in regard to how exercise fits into our lives, there are always opportunities for most of us to improve and enhance our routines. We must use our individual preferences, health status, and learning styles to find an exercise routine that is both challenging and satisfying. Over the course of our lives these habits will likely evolve with our bodies, hopefully to help enhance our daily lives and our health.

CHAPTER 22
NUTRITION

AS WITH MANY OF THE TOPICS we tackle in this book, nutrition deserves its own book entirely if not a whole library to cover it in depth. But since it's only one of many subjects we're discussing in this book, we'll devote this chapter to discussing the most important concepts that we believe hold true and sharing our take on many of the current trends in nutrition. While it is already clear throughout the entirety of this book that we are advocates of supplemental vitamins for many situations, we also believe strongly that good nutrition is the foundation for good health and that there is no substitute for eating a wide variety of fresh healthful foods.

Vitamins are important to fill in the gaps. In today's world there are many gaps, in part because our soil no longer gives our produce the nutrients it once had, our sunscreen and living habits shield us from the sun, and our daily habits preclude our eating an ideal balance of foods all the time. But we should still all attempt to eat well and keep an eye on our health. A 2015 study in the *Journal of the American College of Nutrition* found that over 40 percent of the U.S. adult population had insufficient intake of key micronutrients. Clearly there is some work to be done.

It is safe to say that there are not hard-and-fast rules about the exact correct diet for any one person. We are all individuals, and just as our needs for supplemental vitamins vary from person to person so too does our ideal diet. Taste preferences, allergies, religious observances, schedules, financial situations, access to food, health conditions, and social circumstances influence each of our diets every day. To try to take these factors out of the equation and proclaim a set universal ideal diet would be both unrealistic and foolish. Rather, we should look at the principles that drive healthful eating and find out how each of us can apply them to our own circumstances.

We grew up in the 1970s and '80s learning about the traditional food pyramid, a graphic pyramid-shaped representation of "healthful" eating that was built upon a base of grains. It then stacked on fruits and vegetables, then meats and dairy, and a small summit of oils and sweets. In 2014 the concept of the pyramid was replaced by the USDA with a new icon called MyPlate, a cute visual in which over a quarter of the plate consists of vegetables, a smaller portion is allotted to fruit, and about a quarter is devoted each to grains and meat. The plate is accompanied by a small portion of dairy.

This grand shift in USDA graphics may be representative of a slightly less dramatic shift from a grain-based diet to one that has more emphasis on vegetables. The takeaway is that one half of your plate should be composed mostly of vegetables and some fruit. This is a manifestation of our thinking that a plant-based diet is ideal for most aspects of health—namely, prevention of cancer and heart disease (the leading causes of death in the United States).

Meat has an ever-shrinking spot on the plate. Some nutritionists suggest that while meat was once the central feature of a meal, it has now moved to the role of a condiment. Meaning, it should be a small dressing of sorts for largely vegetable-centric meals. The type of meat—red meat versus "leaner" types, such as chicken or fish (generally an excellent option and a natural source of our beloved omega-3s)—seems to be less of a concern when you eat only a little of it.

A Word on Protein

You probably read the last paragraph about eating minimal meat and asked, "If there is minimal meat in the meal, how should we be getting protein?"

It seems like messages about protein bombard us every day. Protein bars and powders abound. Likewise, many food labels boast a certain number of grams of protein, alluring us to believe, "Well, then it must be healthy." As a society, we seem to have become protein crazed.

But the question remains: Are we really lacking in protein? Actually, most of us are not. The U.S. RDA for protein is 46 grams for women and 56 grams for men. (This is roughly 0.8 grams per kilogram of body weight—in common terms, about one-third of a gram per pound of body weight). Since many foods that we eat contain protein (even for vegetarians and vegans), those grams add up fairly quickly. For example, a yogurt has 11 grams of protein, and a serving of meat has over 20. Dairy products, tofu, eggs, beans, and rice are other common sources.

Of course, we do not all have the same requirements for protein. Because each of us has a different body type, overall diet, exercise routine, and health history, various factors about an individual do influence how much protein they should consume—just as many factors determine what our vitamin needs are.

As outlined above, men and women have slightly different baseline protein requirements. It is generally felt that those in extreme training situations (e.g., marathon running, competitive swimming, etc.) require more protein in their diets. Similarly, people who are recovering from protein deprivation due to illness or a severe burn also need more protein to replenish their stores. However, the vast majority of us (even those who exercise with intensity) are actually getting or exceeding the recommended daily protein intake.

If you are trying to step your fitness regimen up a notch, you will see protein powders galore, boasting they will make you into Miss or Mr. Universe. However when it comes to building muscles by consuming protein, there is clearly a point of diminishing returns. Increasing your protein if you are falling short of your training demands is worth it only to a point. It appears that anything beyond 1.8 g/kg of body weight per day (roughly twice the listed usual U.S. RDA for protein) is no more beneficial for those looking to gain strength or body mass. Sorry to break it to all of you bodybuilders out there who are putting down gallons of protein drinks every day. It's probably not doing much for you, other than adding a lot of calories (which may be okay if you are doing that much exercise).

So, even 0.66 grams of protein per pound of body weight is a very high goal and not necessarily beneficial for building big muscles (if that is even your goal). The question is whether eating too much protein can be harmful. There is conflicting data on this. Some have suggested that diets excessive in protein can be harmful to the kidneys. We do know this to be true in those with existing kidney disease. However, it has not been proven to be so in those with healthy kidneys. It is certainly important to consume enough fluids with protein, because excess protein can deplete you of fluids and this can put stress on the kidneys.

Some data suggest that too much protein intake is associated with higher risks of cancer. However, the study also found this reversed in older age. It also is unclear if the protein itself is raising the cancer risk or if it's the associated animal fat consumption that could be causing the negative effect.

Protein seems to come up a great deal these days in the context of weight loss. Fitness trainers, as well as the food and supplement industry, lead people to believe that the simple act of eating protein must somehow cause weight loss. Not so. Actually, protein can *impede* weight loss because foods high in protein are also rich in calories. This is a natural function of protein being a great source of energy. However, it also is the case that many artificial vehicles for protein (bars, powers, gels, shakes, etc.) have lots of additives that further increase their caloric content. Therefore, do not assume that more protein is always better when you are trying to trim down.

There are some reasons that protein is still very important, even if you are not looking to win the Mr. or Miss Universe competition. Foods high in protein (and fats) tend to be satisfying. They are digested less rapidly than those with lots of carbs, and they do not produce the natural insulin rush that sugary foods do. Therefore, they do not cause major drops in blood levels a few hours later. In other words, proteins satisfy your appetite for longer. Eating protein-based meals and snacks tends to minimize the ravenous hunger that follows eating a quickly digested carb.

For this reason, try to balance your snacks and meals so they contain at least some protein (and remember that doesn't have to be a burger). If you are in intense training, recovering from illness, or you want muscles that Popeye would envy, then push up to twice the RDA for protein (in addition to the actual work that goes into building those muscles). One rule to live by is to aim to get 20–30 percent of your calories from protein. You can calculate the protein calories in something by looking at the grams of protein and multiplying them by four (i.e., each gram of protein has 4 calories, while fats have 9 calories per gram and carbs have 4). The goal is to then find a balance between the three.

Chances are, if you do the math, protein is abundant in your diet. If it is not, look for some natural ways to add it in via eggs, dairy, lean meats, or legumes, rather than artificially produced products. These may have the cachet of "protein," but they may come with other undesirable additives. Just because something contains protein does not mean that it trumps the fact that it is a processed food.

Carbohydrate Confusion

If we had written this book in the mid-1990s, most people wouldn't even have known what a carb is. At that time everyone was so focused on fat-free eating that they didn't realize that the mainstay of their diets were carbohydrates. Fat-free was where it was at, so everyone shoveled in the breads, pastas, and the like. It's hard to believe, but people actually lost weight doing this. Then the fad wore off and the pendulum shifted. Suddenly the Atkins™ diet came into vogue and "no carbs" became the new regime.

Here we stand today, wondering, "Are carbs really that bad?" Carbohydrates are actually an essential part of our diets. They are our best source of quick energy. They also comprise a range of foods, from fruits and vegetables to overly processed bread products to whole grains. Many people believe that all carbohydrates should be banned from the planet, but we do not.

What we do believe is that carbohydrates should be eaten in moderation as part of a thoughtful, balanced diet. The USDA's MyPlate graphic suggests that carbs comprise one quarter of your plate. This is a reasonable rule of thumb. Carbohydrates are not generally rich in other vitamins and nutrients, but the "whole grain" variety and options like brown rice do tend to have more fiber and are thus preferred.

The data on no- or very low-carb diets do suggest that they are superior for weight loss than other diets, in the short term. It is our experience that severe carb restriction is not a sustainable practice, and most people "fall off the wagon" and gain back whatever weight carb restriction may have helped them lose.

Carbohydrates are not the devil in disguise. They do, however, have a limited usefulness in that they are quickly digested and do not tend to satisfy our appetites for long. A normal person's body secretes insulin after eating carbs. This rapidly lowers blood sugar and can then lead to a lower blood sugar and further hunger and/ or fatigue. As a result, carbs do not satisfy us. Because people with elevated blood sugar or full-blown diabetes do not secrete insulin, their circulating levels of sugar are elevated and various organs in their bodies are at risk of damage. For this reason, these people should use caution with carbs, although even they need not eliminate carbs altogether.

Some nutrition experts recommend even those with diabetes have between 45 and 60 grams of carbs per meal, depending on body weight. So even those with the most limited ability to metabolize sugars need some carbohydrates at every meal for optimal metabolism and energy. Those without blood-sugar concerns may be able to handle more, but that is a topic for discussion with your doctor to determine your ideal intake. It should also be noted that there is a difference between simple carbs, such as refined sugar or corn syrup, and complex carbs, such as those that are part of whole foods (which also contain fiber), like fruits and vegetables as well as grains and legumes. Generally speaking, the more fiber paired with a carb, the better, thus the emphasis should be on the complex carbs.

All in all, carbs are part of a healthful diet if kept in moderation and in balance with other healthy food choices. They should be limited, but not feared. And by no means should they be replaced exclusively by a diet excessively high in saturated fats.

The Dairy Dilemma

Dairy products have always been a staple of the Western diet. They play an important role in providing many of us with significant portions of protein, calcium, and B vitamins. Many holistic sources and trendy diets suggest eliminating dairy from the diet. For example, several diets out there advise eliminating dairy because of its role in inflammation. It is true that some people who stop eating dairy see great relief in their symptoms of certain arthritic, inflammatory, and autoimmune conditions. But as with most dietary concerns, it is an individual choice and is certainly not a blanket recommendation. Also, by no means do all people with these conditions find improvement in their symptoms when they stop consuming dairy. If you are plagued by symptoms of inflammatory arthritis (conditions such as rheumatoid arthritis, lupus, and Sjögren's syndrome), IBD (such as Crohn's), asthma, or the like, it's certainly worth giving a dairy-free lifestyle a try. However, if after a few weeks you do not see improvement, it is our feeling that you have no need to abstain from dairy.

Many people stop eating dairy because of lactose intolerance. This diagnosis is a very real condition that plagues many people as they get older. It is more prevalent in non-Caucasian individuals but can be an issue for anyone. Lactose intolerance tends to occur more often later in life, since most children are able to tolerate cow's milk.

Lactose is the form of sugar that is found typically in milk and other dairy products in varying amounts. We all have lactase, an enzyme found in our GI tracts that helps digest lactose. As we age (or sometimes after we have a temporary GI illness, such as a "stomach bug" accompanied by vomiting and diarrhea), many of us experience a decline in our gut lactase levels, which leads to an inability to properly digest lactose and to the resultant symptoms of cramping, gas, bloating, and diarrhea experienced after eating dairy products.

The key to understanding lactose intolerance is to recognize that this condition represents a spectrum, not an all-or-nothing situation. Different people have different tolerances for dairy products. Many people can have milk in cereal in the morning or with coffee and then later in the day have trouble if they push the envelope with another serving of dairy—likely because they have essentially saturated their lactose receptors for the day and used up all their lactase. Some people have very low levels of lactase and experience GI distress from even traces of dairy. Others have trouble with certain whole-milk products, but fewer issues with cheese or yogurt. Again, this is a very individual thing. For this reason, there should be no strict admonishment against eating dairy for those who find an amount they can tolerate. There is no harm in eating dairy if you do not have distress from it, and in fact it remains a great source of calcium and, in the case of yogurt specifically, one of the few easily obtained natural sources of probiotics. These are the good bacteria that help your gut stay in balance. (See the Constipation and IBS chapter for more information both on dairy's role in triggering IBS symptoms and on the benefits of probiotics.)

Especially since people tend to be more restricted with their intake of meat—particularly red meat—today, dairy can be a valued protein source. Though, as a source of animal fat, it too should be consumed in moderation. As of 2014, most sources suggest that plant-based diets (in which the majority of, but not all, food is plant based) are likely to lead to lower rates of cancer, diabetes, and heart disease. Still, who can survive without an occasional ice cream treat? Not us, that's for sure.

The Glory of Gluten-Free

If there's one huge trend in nutrition since the early 2000s, it's gluten-free eating. Gluten-free items are found on restaurant menus, in cookbooks, pharmaceuticals, hair products(!), and more. Even certain paints and craft products have been labeled as such. Perhaps the next frontier will be gluten-free hotel rooms and cars.

We jest about the overabundance of this term, but the origins of its necessity, celiac disease, is no laughing matter. Celiac is an auto-immune condition (often associated with others in this family, such as type 1 diabetes, thyroid disorders, and rheumatoid arthritis) that occurs when eating gluten (not likely washing your hair with it) causes the lining of your small intestine to become inflamed.

The resultant condition can cause a range of symptoms, from GI distress to stunted growth, osteoporosis, and anemia (because of poor absorption of other key nutrients such as vitamin D and iron). Perhaps the most-feared result of untreated celiac disease is an association with GI lymphomas (cancer). For these many reasons, people with diagnosed celiac should avoid gluten at all costs. Even trace amounts in food can lead to negative effects. Celiac is a condition that should be diagnosed first based on bloodwork used as a screening test then confirmed on biopsy via an endoscopy procedure, in which a gastro-enterologist uses a camera scope to actually take a small sample of the lining of your small intestine.

Gluten is found in many foods, typically those containing wheat (pasta, bread, cereal, etc.) but also many other foods such as soy sauce and some salad dressings, among others. Given the range of "gluten-free" products, it can be avoided more easily these days than in the past. However, is there rationale to being strictly gluten-free if you do not have celiac? Medically speaking, generally not. Many people have gluten intolerances (i.e., they get some type of symptoms from eating gluten, including GI upset and arthritic symptoms). These people can abstain from gluten if they feel better doing so. However, it is by no means gospel that anyone with IBS, rheumatoid arthritis, or the like is banished to live gluten-free for all eternity. As with the lactose issue above, an intolerance is exactly that. It is not a potentially life-threatening condition (though celiac is if not treated properly). Therefore, as with abstaining from dairy, our advice is quite similar—try going off it, and see how you feel.

For those who swear by gluten-free because they feel better, it is our recommendation to choose naturally gluten-free foods (generally non-processed real foods such as lean meats, vegetables, and rice will fill the bill). We suggest caution with foods that normally contain gluten that are formulated to be "gluten-free." Typically they are filled with high-fat and sometimes high-sugar substitutes to make up for the flavor or consistency lost with the gluten. So skip the gluten-free pancakes and opt for a Greek yogurt with fruit (that is if you are not also dairy-free).

Only Organic?

Amid the rapidly growing list of food certifications, organic has taken off since the early 2000s. One can find organic labeling on a host of products similar in scope to the gluten-free offerings. Is the hype worth it or in fact true? Yes and no.

Certified organic means the contents have been grown in a manner to meet various criteria. They have been grown without pesticides and on soil that has been free of pesticides for a certain duration of time. Naturally this sounds much better than food that is doused in chemicals to increase its shelf life.

But organic is often synonymous with expensive. The question is whether it is worth the time and effort to ingest primarily organic foods. The answer is sometimes. It is probably worth it for dairy products, at least getting hormone-free milk if you drink it often. Free-range chicken and beef and cage-free eggs are also recommended. All animals that eat more grass than grain (fed to the typical cows and chickens) have higher levels of omega-3s in their meat and their milk. The downside? There is a theoretical risk of more bacterial contamination in food that has fewer preservatives.

Certain produce makes sense to buy organic, typically those items that are sprayed with more pesticides. Examples include berries, apples, potatoes, spinach, and grapes. All fruits and vegetables should be thoroughly washed to rid them of pesticide residues.

Are organic foods more nutrient rich? Unfortunately, this has not been proven. In theory using less chemical fertilizers should ultimately translate into more nutrient-rich soil. The only nutrient so far that appears to be more plentiful in organic produce is phosphorus, which is important for bone building.

As of 2015 another huge buzz phrase in the nutrition world is genetically modified organisms or "GMOs," referring to mostly fruits and vegetables that have been grown from seed with their DNA modified to change certain qualities of the products—i.e., tomatoes that are a darker red or stay useable longer. There is huge controversy over this topic. It makes intuitive sense to think that messing with nature is not good for us and may have unintended consequences. This has not been proven. We are fans of local organically grown produce, so by all means that should be your preferred venue when possible. However the "non-GMO" certification is popping up on everything from salad dressing to cereal, and its significance is uncertain in these contexts. Vous Vitamin® products in fact do proudly bear this certification.

Organic and non-GMO are important considerations. However, as with most things context is king and you better put your time, effort, and dollars into purchasing food products that are healthful and comprise a well-balanced diet rather than boxes that bear seals galore. In fact, less packaged products are generally better for you anyway, so perhaps we should all stop reading so many labels and focus on buying whole-food products that don't have labels at all.

Finicky about Fats

The year 2014 witnessed much upheaval in both the medical community's and the general population's thinking about what fats we should and shouldn't consume. During the preceding decades, there was a significant push to limit fat intake in the name of heart health. The American Heart Association guidelines proposed that limiting fat and cholesterol intake would be the road to healthier hearts for all Americans. This is likely true in part.

The problem is that the recommendation to reduce saturated fat intake (saturated fats are fats found in nature, typically in the form of animal fat from meat or dairy products) led to an uptick in consumption of certain other fats such as hydrogenated fats (these are man-made fats produced to create foods that stay edible longer— think Twinkies™). These fats are used in fried foods and commercial baked goods—typically paired with lots of sugar and carbs. Turns out the same properties that make hydrogenated fats keep food products stable and unchanged are the same properties that cause these fats to settle in your arteries. You can then see how the "less saturated fat" thing might backfire in terms of the subsequent rise in obesity, diabetes, and heart disease. We traded one evil for another.

The early 2000s were marked by a backlash against hydrogenated fats. They were in fact banned from New York City restaurants in 2007 and have additionally been condemned by the FDA. One of the trendier things to boast on food labels lately is "No trans fats." It's a good thing to boast. So clearly trans fats are passé. But what about the other fats?

The polyunsaturated fats found in many natural, non-meat-based foods seem to be the healthiest of all fats—in things like olive oil; the oil found in fatty fishes, like salmon; and nuts and avocados. These are known to raise HDL, or "good," cholesterol (see the Cholesterol chapter for more information) and are the staples of the Mediterranean diet, based largely on lots of fish, vegetables, and limited whole grains and touted for its heart-healthy effects. However, a 2014 study in the *Annals of Internal Medicine* suggests that there may not be a huge difference between saturated and unsaturated fats in their effects on heart health.

There is more research to be done for sure. It is our belief that some saturated fat is okay, though the less meat-based, more plant-focused Mediterranean diet is preferable. The key is not to cut out the carbs altogether and dive into the saturated fats (as was trendy with the Atkins diet, in which many adherents eliminated carbs completely and then feasted on bacon all day). As we have said before finding balance is optimal, and in this case the balance should favor lean meats and fish, lots of veggies, and the intermittent smaller portion of red meat and (more complex) carbs.

For certain, more remains to be learned about the exact link between fats, carbs, and subsequent diabetes and heart disease. It is safe to say that the pattern that we have seen emerge from all of these findings about diet and disease is that the less manipulated the foods are the healthier they seem to be (i.e., the hydrogenated oils are worse than most of the natural sources for oil. Likewise whole grains are healthier carbs than highly refined ones. The guiding principle should then be to avoid overprocessed or engineered foods. Starting with good raw ingredients, you should create the food you eat. As they say, shop the perimeter of the grocery store (produce, meats, fish, and dairy) and skip the aisles full of cans and boxes and you will be safe. You will also manage to avoid a lot of unhealthy sodium and other additives.

Nutrition may sound complicated. However, it is our belief that back to basics is the way to go. That is, eat simple (typically unpackaged) foods and you will do well. Instead of fixating on measuring every gram of protein or carb, focus on a healthy variety and balance of ingredients, and you will meet most of your body's needs. Vitamins can then be used to fill in the gaps.

PART FIVE:
FINAL THOUGHTS

A FEW THINGS BEFORE WE GO

THROUGHOUT THIS BOOK, we have tried to provide a balanced perspective on a variety of health topics and the ways in which vitamins can be used safely and effectively to better your health. While supplements are not a be-all and end-all cure for every medical condition, they often play a very useful role in both preventing and treating disease. They can supplement many common medications to help treat various conditions, or they can be used in the context of other lifestyle changes to both prevent and treat ailments, as well as to help people minimize the use of prescription drugs.

However, our needs for specific vitamins can vary greatly from person to person. We are not all the same—we do not eat the same, live the same, or have the same health problems or complaints—so, not surprisingly, we all have individual vitamin needs.

Our company, Vous Vitamin®, came into being based on this premise. We felt like we were seeing patient after patient confused about what they should or should not take. Many wanted to use vitamins as a part of their health-care plan but did not know how best to do so. Some had problems that could be solved with vitamins that they did not even know about before seeing us. As physicians, we recognize that each patient had his or her own story to tell, and our recommendations vary based on those details.

We created the concept of the Personalized Multivitamin™ and then we produced the products that we felt met the standards of quality and purity that we had been searching for. We crafted an online diagnostic survey and computerized algorithm to ensure that each person got a product that met their needs. We also set out to educate our consumers and dispel many of the common misconceptions about vitamins and health that we hear from friends and patients every day. We started blogging to provide people with relevant, medically sound information about a wide variety of health topics and the safe and proper use of vitamins.

This book is largely an outgrowth of that blog. Figuring out who will benefit from what vitamin is a great challenge, but we hope that in these pages you have found information that pertains to your specific health needs. To continue to learn the most up-to-date information from our continued blog posts, visit our Vous Vitamin Blog. We would love to hear back from you as well about your own experiences with vitamins.

—Arielle and Romy

VITAMIN GLOSSARY

THE BULK OF OUR BOOK has covered various conditions and their treatment and/or prevention. We have addressed a number of vitamins and supplements over the course of the book and the roles they can play for different people depending on their individual dietary and health needs. A number of essential nutrients appear frequently. We have created a glossary of many of the vitamins to act as a quick-reference guide for readers who are curious about the ins and outs and pros and cons of specific common vitamins. This glossary is by no means an exhaustive list of every vitamin or supplement we have mentioned or that is commercially available; rather, it features the highlights. As always, each of the following vitamins should be taken in the context of the individual's circumstances.

A Is for Awful

In our journey to learn about vitamins, perhaps one of the first eye-opening findings we had was regarding vitamin A. Taking too much vitamin A can potentially cause great harm. We hear so much about why we should take vitamin A, when it has the potential to cause a number of problems. In fact, for a while it was commonplace for eye doctors to dole out large doses of vitamin A for "eye health." There is some basis for this, but more on it later.

Vitamin A sounds so compelling. It is one of the vitamins that bear the cachet of being an "antioxidant." This class of vitamins helps the body clear toxic free radicals and stop damage to cells, theoretically helping reduce cancer and heart disease. What could be bad about this?

On a broad scale, it is probably true that antioxidants do some of these great things. However, that does not necessarily mean that taking large amounts of supplemental vitamin A (as most standard multivitamins contain) will actually have that intended effect. In fact, the opposite may occur. Taking the wrong amounts of certain supplements may actually increase rates of cancer. It's true! The theory behind vitamin A is great, but the reality (as shown by the scientific data) proves otherwise. You have to be careful with these products—even if they are sold over the counter.

As it turns out, vitamin A (consisting of both retinol and beta-carotene) is found in many fruits and vegetables in moderate amounts. Very few people in developed countries lack in this vitamin. Those living in extreme poverty or in the developing world do often have vitamin A deficiency, which can cause blindness. However, most of us eating a typical diet in the United States are far from deficient in this vitamin. Remember your mother telling you to eat your carrots so you can see better? She did know a little something. But most of us actually are doing pretty well as far as obtaining vitamin A from our diet.

Too much of a good thing is not always better. In looking at the medical research, it seems that taking supplemental vitamin A really does little good and, in fact, may cause harm. Several studies showed that people who took supplemental vitamin A had significantly higher risks of cancer—principally lung cancer (but also prostate cancer in men). Likewise, some studies looking at the impact on heart disease show little benefit to vitamin A supplementation, and perhaps harm.

On top of that, higher vitamin A intake also has been shown to greatly increase rates of osteopenia (decreased bone density) and hip fractures in women. Although many touted vitamin A supplementation as useful for preventing cataracts and macular degeneration, many large trials have shown no benefit to supplementing vitamin A in this arena either. It may turn out that certain other vitamins, similar but not the same as vitamin A, such as lutein and lycopene could have a role in eye health and cancer prevention.

Ironically, most standard multivitamins contain exceedingly high doses of vitamin A—sometimes up to five times the U.S. RDA (which is 700–900 mcg daily). Taking these high doses for long periods of time is sure to allow vitamin A to accumulate in your body. It is a fat-soluble vitamin, which means it is primarily stored in the liver and does not leave your body quickly. This is part of the reason we are not often deficient in it in this part of the world: If we eat a few foods high in vitamin A, we can store this vitamin for a very long time.

Overdosing on vitamin A can in the short term lead to a syndrome called hypervitaminosis A in which people not only turn yellow, but also experience severe headaches, skin irritation, and, in extreme cases, coma or death.

We find it disturbing that many off-the-shelf multivitamins contain several times the U.S. RDA for vitamin A, when these are the doses shown to have caused many of these problems. Don't get us wrong, if you are vitamin A deficient (as many children in Africa and other developing countries are) you should by all means take supplements to help protect your vision and immunity. However, if you live in the U.S. and eat a decent variety of foods, you are very unlikely to need much in the way of vitamin A (and certainly not megadoses as many vitamins contain).

So what about your mother imploring you to eat carrots to improve your eyesight? We agree with her. Stop the madness of high-dose supplements and get your vitamin A the way nature intended you to, by eating a healthful and balanced diet. It takes just a minimal amount of fruit or vegetables to meet the U.S. RDA of vitamin A. Plus vitamin A is a fat-soluble vitamin, meaning once you take some it actually stays with you for months (your fat cells hold on to it). So, eat your carrots and take only the supplements you need, not those that could be potentially harmful.

Vitamin A Highlights

What It Does
Helps with vision, immunity, and cell growth

Where It's Found
Meat, dairy, veggies (red peppers, carrots, spinach, and broccoli to name a few), fruits, and fortified cereals

Daily Dose
5,000 IUs

Can Be Used For
Improving vision and immune health, and has "antioxidant" properties, such as fighting inflammation

What Happens If You Are Deficient?
Profound deficiency can lead to blindness and low immunity

What Happens If You Take Too Much?
Some evidence of higher rates of cancer, osteoporosis, yellow skin, and coma if severe

B All You Can B

There are a number of B vitamins, some of which also go by other names. Going in numerical order, we will begin with B1. Also known as thiamine, this essential vitamin is just that—essential. If you become deficient in thiamine, you can become gravely ill. This can happen quickly since it is a water-soluble vitamin that is not stored in our cells for long. People who are profoundly deficient in thiamine get severe neurological consequences, leading to brain damage (most commonly seen in late-stage alcoholics). Severe thiamine deficiency is also seen in the malnourished in developing countries (at which point it is called beriberi) and can cause severe gastrointestinal symptoms and skin diseases.

In the developed world, we get thiamine through many foods, such as beef, milk, and legumes. However, many of us do not consume much of the above, and even if we do, we may not get quite enough. Therefore, optimal neurological and GI health may be achieved with some extra thiamine. Since alcohol consumption seems to deplete our stores of this vital substance, repleting it is essential if you enjoy a glass of wine or cocktail from time to time.

Frequent alcohol use can deplete your B1 stores. For this and other reasons (such as breast cancer risk and heart health), women are advised not to have more than an average of one drink per day. The recommendation for men is not more than an average of two drinks daily. Some choose to spread these drinks out over a week's time, while others like to do it up with several drinks on a weekend. Regardless, keep stock of your habits. If you feel you have a problem with alcohol consumption, please reach out to your health-care professional.

In the hospital setting, when a person comes in acutely intoxicated it is standard care to give them what is called a "banana bag." This is a bright yellow IV solution that contains a variety of vitamins including B1. It is given to prevent some of the neurological consequences of excessive alcohol. At Vous Vitamin®, we realized that we could learn something from this practice and we created our Recovery Act Situational Supplement™. This is a tablet that is composed of the same components found in the banana bag. It is intended to be taken when consuming alcohol to help minimize feeling poorly the next day. Our customers rave about it.

If you just like to have a few drinks with friends here and there, cheers! You may actually be reducing your risk of heart disease, and as long as you don't exceed that seven or fourteen-per-week maximum (depending on your sex), studies show you are not increasing your risk of breast cancer. Just make sure to drink responsibly, which includes not only finding a designated driver, but also ensuring that you supplement your habit appropriately. A daily multivitamin tailored to your needs may be in order as most multivitamins include thiamine in some amount. That's the lowdown on thiamine (B1). As for the others in this family of vitamins, that will have to "B" continued . . .

Vitamin B1 (Thiamine) Highlights

What It Does
Involved in nerve function and digestive health

Where It's Found
Grains, beans, nuts, and meat

Daily Dose
1.1–1.4 mg

Can Be Used For (in Higher Doses)
Alcohol intoxication and GI health

What Happens If You Are Deficient?
Trouble with brain function and memory, GI disturbances, and menstrual cramps

What Happens If You Take Too Much?
Rare side effects; extreme overdoses can cause low blood pressure

Vitamin B2: 2B or Not to B

Vitamin B2 is also known as riboflavin. This essential vitamin plays a role in converting carbohydrates to energy. Like other B vitamins it is an antioxidant vitamin, meaning it helps fight damaging particles in the body. It plays a role in growth and blood cell formation.

Most Americans are not deficient in this vitamin since it is found in a great variety of food sources. Some typical foods that contain it are yeast, almonds, grains, rice, mushrooms, dairy products, eggs, and vegetables such as spinach and broccoli. However, those who are deficient can experience symptoms such as fatigue, skin issues (such as cracking around the mouth), and slowed growth.

The U.S. RDA for B2 is 1.1–1.6 mg daily depending on age and stage of life. In addition to food sources B2 can be found in some multivitamins, fortified cereals, and B-complex vitamins. It often comes in tabs of 25, 50, or 100 mg.

It has been suggested that riboflavin supplementation may decrease cataract formation. More research is needed. However, it should be noted that if one takes more than 10 mg of riboflavin daily, he or she can get eye damage from the sun. Thus, you should use extreme caution and wear sunglasses when outside if you take supplemental B2.

Riboflavin in high doses (400 mg daily) has also been studied as a means to successfully reduce migraine frequency. The mechanism for this is unknown, but it is a reasonable thing to try in those who suffer frequent migraines. However, as mentioned above, eye protection should be worn in the sun.

Vitamin B2 (Riboflavin) Highlights

What It Does

Helps convert carbohydrates to energy

Where It's Found

Yeast, whole grains, eggs, dairy, and vegetables

Daily Dose

1.1–1.6 mg

Can Be Used for (in Higher Doses)

Depression, PMS symptoms, and migraine headaches

What Happens If You Are Deficient?

Fatigue, skin problems, and slow growth

What Happens If You Take Too Much?

Sun-damaged eyes and itchy skin

B3: Niacin Is Not So Nice

Vitamin B3, more commonly known as niacin (or nicotinamide) has been much talked about over the years. Like other B vitamins, it plays an important role in the body's use of energy. Specifically, niacin also plays a role in various hormones produced by the adrenal glands, and high doses of niacin seem to affect serum lipid (cholesterol) levels.

Vitamin B3 deficiency is rare in the United States, though it can occur in alcoholics and those with digestive diseases. It is more often seen in the developing world. In the United States we get niacin through a variety of food sources, including yeast, beef, various kinds of fish, and beets. Also, many of our breads and cereals are fortified with niacin. In addition, foods that contain tryptophan, such as eggs and poultry, are naturally converted to niacin in our bodies. The U.S. RDA for niacin is 14–17 mg daily for adults. This is not hard to come by.

Those deficient in niacin (rarely seen here) get a syndrome called pellagra, taught to every medical student as the three Ds: dementia (memory loss), diarrhea, and dermatitis (a scaling, red skin rash). Milder deficiency can cause fatigue, depression, and vomiting. These deficiencies can be seen in those with GI absorption issues, namely Crohn's disease and colitis, or after major intestinal surgeries, such as gastric bypass. Deficiency can be remedied relatively quickly, since B3 is a water-soluble vitamin and levels rise rapidly with modest doses of replacement.

Much higher doses of niacin have been used to treat cholesterol issues. Niacin does in fact lower LDL (bad cholesterol), lower triglycerides (also undesirable), and raise HDL levels (good cholesterol). Sound too good to be true? It is. Several 2014 studies from the *New England Journal of Medicine* examine niacin's effects. The conclusion that can be drawn is that, while the cholesterol numbers improve, the outcomes of stroke and heart attack do not improve significantly with niacin. (For a more in-depth discussion, see the Cholesterol chapter.)

In addition to not having the intended effects on cardiovascular disease, niacin can have a tremendous number of side effects. We have always known that people experience terrible flushing reactions with high-dose niacin (though these can sometimes be avoided by taking aspirin beforehand). In addition niacin has been known to raise blood sugars, prompting worse control in diabetics and even increasing the risk of developing diabetes in some who use it. Perhaps most concerning is the potential for serious liver damage with niacin. This was also documented in the *New England Journal of Medicine* and is something we have witnessed in our own practices when people have used very high doses (over 100 mg daily).

In short, we do not endorse the use of high-dose niacin. Rather, it is best found in natural foods and fortified foods in moderate doses.

B3 (Niacin) Highlights

What It Does

Helps the body use energy, creates certain hormones, and regulates cholesterol

Where It's Found

Fish, beets, yeast, and fortified cereals and breads

Daily Dose

14–17 mg

Can Be Used for (in Higher Doses)

Treating cholesterol

What Happens If You Are Deficient?

Diarrhea, fatigue, memory trouble, and skin problems

What Happens If You Take Too Much?

Flushing, high blood sugar, and liver damage

Vitamin B6: Six of One, Half a Dozen of the Other

Vitamin B6, also called pyridoxine, is an essential water-soluble vitamin. It is useful in making antibodies (part of immunity), neurotransmitters (chemicals that regulate mood in the brain), processing proteins, keeping blood sugar normal, making hemoglobin (part of red blood cells), and regulating nerve function.

In the United States, B6 deficiency is rare. The U.S. RDA is 1.3–1.7 mg daily. It is found in many dietary sources, including bananas, avocado, meat and poultry, grains, and legumes. When deficiencies are present, the effects include neurological symptoms such as depression, confusion, irritability, and some skin rashes. At Vous Vitamin®, we included B6 in our Power Up Situational Supplement™, which is intended for occasional use for exercise or an intense day. The focus of the supplement is on energy, and an extra burst of B6 when you need it can be very helpful.

B6 can often be supplemented via a multivitamin or a B-complex vitamin. Excess doses may cause numbness or difficulty coordinating movement.

B6 (Pyridoxine) Highlights

What It Does
Helps process proteins and makes neurotransmitters (helps brain with mood)

Where It's Found
Bananas, grains, meat and poultry, and legumes

Daily Dose
1.3–1.7 mg

Can Be Used for (in Higher Doses)

Migraine and cataract prevention

What Happens If You Are Deficient?

Neurological symptoms, skin rash, and anemia

What Happens If You Take Too Much?

Tingling and trouble coordinating movement

B7: Biotin for Thin Hair

Biotin or vitamin B7 (previously called vitamin H) has gotten much acclaim for its role in hair and nail growth. It helps with the use of proteins, carbohydrates, and fats and the synthesis of certain proteins used by the body for growth. This seems to play an important part in creating keratin for healthy hair and nail formation.

Biotin deficiency is hard to diagnose since blood levels cannot be checked. Rather, it is a clinical diagnosis based on symptoms such as thinning hair, brittle nails, and sometimes fatigue and a scaling rash.

Biotin is found in many common foods such as cauliflower, mushrooms, and dairy products. However, sometimes we do not absorb it adequately. Certain other food ingredients (such as avidin, found in egg whites) actually interfere with its absorption. Thus, supplementing biotin at higher than recommended daily doses can be useful.

The U.S. RDA for biotin is 30–100 mcg. However, recommended dosing of biotin to treat thinning hair is up to 2,500 mcg daily. There appear to be few side effects from taking too much biotin, though some suggest that if it is not taken with other B vitamins (such as folic acid, B12, and B1) your balance of B vitamins can become upset. It is also important to recognize other potential causes of thinning hair or brittle nails (low iron and vitamin D deficiency) and treat them concurrently.

Biotin Highlights

What It Does
Helps build certain body proteins such as keratin

Where It's Found
Cauliflower, mushrooms, dairy products, and egg yolks

Daily Dose
30–100 mcg

Can Be Used for (in Higher Doses)

Hair growth, nail growth, and neuropathy

What Happens If You Are Deficient?

Hair thinning, brittle nails, fatigue, and rashes

What Happens If You Take Too Much?

Imbalance of other B vitamins (if not taking other B vitamins)

B12 Is Important for a Dozen Reasons

Of all the B vitamins, the most common deficiency we see in practice is that of B12. B12 deficiency can be a life-changing problem. Also called cobalamin, this essential vitamin is needed for proper function of the nervous system. Its role in energy conversion of carbohydrates makes nerves function optimally.

Unlike many of the other B vitamins, B12 deficiency is seen commonly in clinical practice in the United States. B12 is found in a number of common foods, namely dairy products, meat, and fish. However, many people do not seem to absorb it adequately. This seems to occur more as people get older and in people taking certain medications (such as the proton-pump inhibitors for acid reflux or metformin for diabetes). We also see lack of absorption after gastric bypass surgery or with some gastrointestinal illnesses. Commonly we find B12 deficiency in people who keep a vegan or vegetarian diet. There is also a small set of people who develop an autoimmune process by which they make antibodies to the stomach cells that typically help absorb B12. This pernicious anemia is associated with other autoimmune illness.

The symptoms of B12 deficiency can be very disturbing. Because of B12's role in the nervous system, symptoms of deficiency typically include neurological complaints. People can suffer from memory loss, numbness and tingling, motor weakness, fatigue, and attention-related issues, among other things, if they are lacking in B12. We have seen a number of people with symptoms resembling multiple sclerosis, Alzheimer's, and other conditions, who have turned out to have B12 deficiency. Their symptoms improved with adequate replacement of B12. Vitamin B12 levels can be checked via bloodwork. However, the blood level for B12 is not always sensitive enough to detect low levels.

B12 can be replaced through pills (commonly combined with other B vitamins or as a multivitamin), nasal sprays, or shots. We find that most mild deficiencies can be rectified with pills, but those with severe deficiencies require shots (at least initially) to build back their levels. Still, it can take a number of months to build up sufficient B12 levels and reverse any of the symptoms experienced with deficiency. At Vous Vitamin®, we included B12 in our Power Up Situational Supplement™, a blend of important electrolytes and vitamins for use when you need an extra boost for a workout or a taxing day. We also incorporate it into many of our multivitamin preparations, because B12 deficiency is common.

Vitamin B12 is perhaps the most common B deficiency and the most important one that we see in everyday practice. There is little downside to replacing it, even in higher doses. We believe that many people can benefit from replacing B12 in varying amounts.

B12 (Cobalamin) Highlights

What It Does

Helps nerves function and helps the body create energy

Where It's Found

Meat, poultry, and dairy

Daily Dose

2.4–2.8 mcg is the U.S. RDA, though many people seem to need higher doses to absorb adequate amounts

Can Be Used for (in Higher Doses)

Energy, attention, memory, and nerve pain

What Happens If You Are Deficient?

Numbness, tingling, memory troubles, and fatigue

What Happens If You Take Too Much?

Allergic reaction in those allergic to cobalt and rashes

Vitamin C: See What It Can Do for You

Vitamin C (also known as ascorbic acid) has gone in and out of style many times over the years. It was brought to the limelight in the 1950s by the chemist Dr. Linus Pauling, who believed vitamin C's effects to be earth shattering. However, it was known way back in the 1700s that English shipmen would get scurvy (the result of vitamin C deficiency) if they didn't consume citrus fruits. They would get bleeding gums, tooth and hair loss, bleeding under the skin, and joint pains if they didn't have any of this vital nutrient while at sea. Thus vitamin C's benefits were understood in some fashion long before Dr. Pauling's era.

According to Dr. Pauling, this antioxidant is the wonder vitamin. He believed it cured the common cold and treated heart disease alike. He was perhaps overzealous about vitamin C, but his beliefs may have been grounded in reality. There is some data to suggest that vitamin C can at least help shorten the duration of the common cold if not prevent it all together (see the Immunity chapter). Its role in heart disease remains unproven, though some theorize that its antioxidant properties should help scavenge the "free radicals" that play a part in this. Likewise, it may help arthritis in part due to this anti-inflammatory effect, but also due to its role in collagen production (creating the cartilage that arthritis destroys).

Vitamin C plays an important role in the absorption of iron, helping the GI tract take in iron properly. Thus, it should be a part of the treatment in any iron-replacement plan. This can be done with a supplement or with food containing relatively high doses (such as a glass of orange juice) taken with the iron pills. At Vous Vitamin®, the iron in any of our products is also paired with vitamin C.

Is there such a thing as too much vitamin C? Absolutely. Useful as it can be, too much is not a good thing. Vitamin C is very acidic (not surprisingly given it is also known as ascorbic acid) and thus can do a number on your stomach in high doses, causing abdominal pain, nausea, and diarrhea. It is also known to cause kidney stones in excessive doses. We believe a fair guideline is not to consume more than

1,000 mg daily. A nice daily supplement should include about 250 mg. However, when coming down with a respiratory infection, taking an extra 250 mg may be useful in boosting immunity.

Vitamin C (Ascorbic Acid) Highlights

What It Does

Helps with synthesis of collagen (part of blood vessels, teeth, hair, and skin)

Where It's Found

Citrus fruits, strawberries, and red peppers

Daily Dose

250 mg

Can Be Used for (in Higher Doses)

Arthritis, iron absorption, hair and nail growth, and immunity

What Happens If You Are Deficient?

Thinning hair, bleeding gums, easy bleeding, and teeth falling out

What Happens If You Take Too Much?

Heartburn, diarrhea, kidney stones, and vomiting

The Calcium Conversation

Calcium is the most abundant mineral in the body. It is essential for blood-vessel function, muscle contraction, and nerve functions since it plays an important role in regulating the way cells work. However, much of the body's calcium is not used for these functions, but instead is stored in the bones and teeth. The body continually draws upon the calcium stored in bones to carry out other functions, when needed. For this reason and for maintaining strong bones, having enough calcium is key.

Until recently, we were doling out calcium supplements for women as if they were candy. The intention was good: Calcium builds bones. Bone density declines with age, so as women are living longer, osteoporosis has reached epidemic proportions. Therefore, it makes sense that we should do anything we can to prevent or minimize this troublesome condition (see the Bone Health chapter for more information). But there is a definite downside to too much calcium.

Previous recommendations included calcium supplements of 1,200–1,500 mg per day. These supplements usually came in the form of large, difficult-to-swallow tablets that were supposed to be taken multiple times daily with food. Beyond the hassle factor, other downsides to taking calcium supplements include unwanted side effects such as upset stomach, kidney stones, constipation, and, less commonly, serious overdoses with high blood levels of calcium. All of that aside, more than half of older women in the U.S. are taking these supplements in the hope of preserving bone density.

However, taking calcium supplements may cause harm. There could be more unintended problems with ingesting large amounts of calcium supplements. The calcium may not just make its way to your bones—it may deposit other places in your body. The most concerning deposits may occur in important blood vessels that supply your heart and brain. This circulating calcium may actually clog arteries and contribute to heart disease and stroke. However, the data still is not definitive and continues to be tested. There is a lot more to be learned. In 2014 a large study suggested that calcium supplements may not lead to greater cardiovascular mortality. A sensible approach to preserving your bones would say that megadoses of calcium supplements may not be the best idea—but dietary calcium still is important.

There are many great sources from which you can get your daily calcium in addition to the commonly thought of milk, cheese, and yogurt. Green leafy vegetables, such as kale, spinach, and broccoli, or even nuts and seeds, such as sesame seeds, almonds, and chickpeas, are all good sources. Most of us can cobble together 1,000 mg or so daily via all of these food sources.

We may still need to take a small amount of calcium supplement. But gone are the days of the big calcium pills. Each person should find the right supplement for their individual needs (the big milk drinker may need less than the lactose-intolerant person). There has been much discussion about which form of calcium is superior to supplement. Calcium carbonate is more commonly found, though some supplements contain calcium citrate. Carbonate is better absorbed with food while citrate is absorbed with or without food. However, no supplemental calcium is useful or absorbed at doses greater than 500 mg at a time. It is our belief that concentrating on food sources with calcium spread throughout the day is first priority, and then a small amount of supplemental calcium can be added if needed.

Vitamin D is very important to calcium absorption and utilization. Additionally, magnesium plays a role in calcium balance in the body. Calcium is an essential mineral that should not be disregarded; however, it should be taken as a supplement only in proper doses and context, and should also be a primary focus in a balanced diet.

Calcium Highlights

What It Does
Regulates cell channels for blood vessel, muscle, and nerve function; builds bones and teeth

Where It's Found
Dairy products, almonds, dark green vegetables, and chickpeas

Daily Dose
1,000–1,500 mg

Can Be Used For (in Higher Doses)
Improving bone density

What Happens If You Are Deficient?
Osteoporosis, weak muscles, and neurological issues

What Happens If You Take Too Much?
Nausea, vomiting, kidney stones, and mental changes

D Is for Delightful

If you read the contents of this book, you are on to the fact that we are big fans of vitamin D. It turns out that it is a vitamin that is incredibly important and its deficiency is exceedingly common. Where we practice in the Chicago area, vitamin D deficiency is the rule more than the exception.

We have known for years that vitamin D is essential for bone health and development. The disease known as rickets is due to profound vitamin D deficiency in childhood. People used to get bowed legs from poor bone growth. Luckily, due to the advent of fortified milk, this condition is now rare. Milk supplies us with small amounts of D, which is better than nothing (about 50 IUs per serving). It is enough to prevent rickets, but not nearly enough to get most of us the amounts of D we need to have normal blood levels of this essential vitamin.

Not surprisingly then, milder forms of vitamin D deficiency are rampant. Vitamin D deficiency may cause bone problems and other symptoms. Without adequate vitamin D, we do not absorb and metabolize calcium properly, and our bones can lose density. Therefore, inadequate vitamin D levels contribute to osteoporosis and the resultant fractures. It is essential to bone development and the prevention of bone loss that we have enough vitamin D. Bone development peaks in our mid-30s, so getting proper amounts of this nutrient in our younger years is imperative. However, its importance continues after bone density peaks and then starts to decline. Adequate vitamin D levels aids bones in maintaining their strength (see our Bone Health chapter for more information).

We first looked at vitamin D because of its role in bone health, but as new research comes out, we are learning that it has many other important roles. Muscles, too, rely on vitamin D to function optimally. People with inadequate vitamin D levels do not have the same muscle strength as those who have enough. Elderly people with low vitamin D levels are much more prone to falls. It is believed that younger people benefit from adequate vitamin D levels as well for both muscle building and general muscle health. Many people report they have fewer tendencies to strain muscles and tendons once they achieve optimal levels of vitamin D. (See the Body Aches chapter.)

In addition to muscle health, vitamin D plays a role in immunity, diabetes prevention, fighting depression, fertility, migraine, and memory. (See the chapters on the aforementioned topics for more information.)

When it comes to taking vitamin D, it turns out that many or most of us need to supplement our diets.

Where does vitamin D come from? Very few natural foods contain it. The only foods that contain it in significant amounts are wild-caught salmon (not farm raised, as most salmon are that we eat) and beef liver. Many foods are fortified with low levels of vitamin D, such as milk, yogurt, and some orange juices. However, a glass of milk has only about 100 IUs of vitamin D, which is a small fraction of the approximate 1,000 IUs we believe most of us need.

The other main source of vitamin D is sunlight. To obtain vitamin D from the sun, we have to have direct sun exposure and not be wearing protective clothing or sunscreen (this may be ill-advised given skin-cancer risks). We absorb vitamin D through our skin, but we must then metabolize it in our liver and kidneys (both must function optimally for this) to transform it into its active form. Complicated, yes?

Long story short, very few of us are managing to do all of this enough in order to get what we need. Therefore, most of us should be taking some form of vitamin D supplement. How much to take varies depending on your individual health history and lifestyle. For example, those who don't absorb as much through diet (those with celiac or IBD) or via the sun (those in northern latitudes) may need more than others. Most daily supplement recommendations range from 400 to 2,000 IUs.

But not just any vitamin D supplement will do—you must get a quality supplement that contains not just vitamin D, but vitamin D3. This is the vitamin's most active form. Unconverted vitamin D is less active, requiring more steps to metabolize it, and is less likely to raise blood levels significantly.

It is also essential you get the correct amount for your needs. This can be determined by your doctor, measuring blood levels, or either of those combined with an analysis of your diet and health habits. At Vous Vitamin® when creating our Personalized Multivitamins™, we ask detailed questions in our diagnostic survey to determine how much vitamin D people need based on their diets, where they live, and other conditions they may have.

Recent data suggest that both too little and too much vitamin D can have detrimental effects. Some studies showed higher rates of cancer with extremely high blood levels. There may also be an increase in inflammatory markers, such as C-reactive protein, at higher blood levels. Physical symptoms of toxic levels are rare, but possible. Kidney stones can form. See Vitamin Horror Stories about how vitamin D toxicity can in fact be life threatening. Vitamin D is a fat-soluble vitamin, meaning it is stored in your body fat and therefore takes a long time to leave your system once it builds up. It also can take six to twelve months to appropriately build up vitamin D stores. Slow and steady wins the race!

Vitamin D Highlights

What It Does
Helps calcium absorption and white blood cell functioning

Where It's Found
Wild-caught salmon, liver, sunlight, and, in small amounts, fortified products

Daily Dose
The U.S. RDA is 400–800 IUs, but many people need higher doses to maintain normal serum levels

Can Be Used for (in Higher Doses)
Osteoporosis, hair loss, migraines, arthritis, and muscle aches

What Happens If You Are Deficient?
Bone loss, thinning hair, fatigue, muscle aches, low energy, and depression

What Happens If You Take Too Much?
High calcium levels, constipation, mental status changes, nausea, vomiting, calcification of blood vessels, and kidney stones

Vitamin E Is for Enigmatic

Vitamin E is both everywhere and enigmatic. At various times in the past, vitamin E has been suggested to be useful for everything from heart disease to dementia prevention to wound healing and more. Thus it appears everywhere in the medical literature regarding vitamins and health. However—and here is where the enigma comes into play—vitamin E seems to play a role in some of these things, yet probably not as much as once thought.

A fat-soluble vitamin and one of the antioxidants, vitamin E is speculated to play some role in reducing inflammation. The mechanism may be the scavenging of toxic free radicals (which are known to cause cellular and DNA damage). Vitamin E's role in cancer prevention has been researched extensively, but the conclusions have been uniformly disappointing. In fact, some studies have shown that higher doses of vitamin E may have some increased incidence of certain cancers, such as prostate cancer in men.

Likewise, studies of vitamin E for prevention of heart disease and stroke have shown little promise. It is fairly evident that vitamin E does cause reduced coagulation and therefore increases bleeding risk. It should be taken in higher doses with caution also for this reason. People on blood thinners should be particularly careful. Most surgeons recommend stopping supplemental vitamin E a week before any procedures are planned to avoid excessive bleeding. This effect may be helpful for those at risk for blood clots as vitamin E may have some role in prevention. Further studies need to be conducted to confirm this.

Vitamin E has been studied for its role in preventing dementia. But again, the outcomes have been unexciting. To the extent that inflammation and clotting may play a role in this disease process, vitamin E may be helpful.

Likewise, there may be a role for vitamin E in treating arthritis, again due to its anti-inflammatory properties. Likely lower doses will suffice for this.

Some large studies have shown that high-dose vitamin E supplementation is associated with higher mortality. For this reason, among others, we believe that high-dose supplementation with vitamin E (anything over 400 IUs per day) is not recommended. There may be some benefit to lower doses, however, for their anti-inflammatory effect.

All in all, vitamin E seems to play a role in many bodily processes. However, rarely does taking large doses seem to have any benefit, and it clearly can have risks. For this reason, we are generally advocates of using vitamin E sparingly. A low dose can be a part of a good multivitamin, but beyond that its use should be limited.

Vitamin E Highlights

What It Does
Protects cell membranes and helps scavenge free radicals

Where It's Found
Vegetable oils, nuts, and green vegetables

Daily Dose
15–19 mg

Can Be Used for (in Higher Doses)
Immunity, memory, blood thinning, and arthritis

What Happens If You Are Deficient?
Muscle weakness, eye problems, and trouble walking

What Happens If You Take Too Much?
Excess bleeding, including cerebral hemorrhage

Folic Acid Is No Folly

Folic acid or folate is a B vitamin (B9) that typically escapes using the B name. It is an essential nutrient that, like other B vitamins, plays a role in energy and metabolism. Folic acid is the synthetic form of the naturally occurring folate. Because folate is found readily in many vegetables and grains, the typical American has many opportunities to eat it. However, this is perhaps not done as much as it should be. Deficiency is associated with those who do not eat enough fruits and vegetables, those who drink large quantities of alcohol, and people with digestive diseases such as Crohn's or celiac disease, which can impair absorption of this vitamin.

Folic acid is most commonly acclaimed for its importance in the developing fetus. There is a well-known association between low folate intake in the pregnant mother and the development of neural tube or spinal cord defects in the developing fetus (i.e., spina bifida, which can be severely debilitating and life threatening). Thus, it is recommended that all women who are pregnant or planning to conceive should ensure adequate folate or folic acid intake, if possible several months in advance of conception.

Folic acid deficiency can manifest with anemia. The red blood cells can appear large in size on a blood count (as they do with B12 deficiency). Symptoms of deficiency can include memory trouble, numbness, tingling, and fatigue. Replacing folic acid can reverse all of these problems. However, it is essential to also rule out B12 deficiency when someone has folic acid deficiency. This is because replacing only the folic acid can partially mask the findings of B12 deficiency so that it goes undetected, but it still causes serious problems (see more under B12).

B9 (Folic Acid) Highlights

What It Does
Useful in energy and development of certain cells (red cells and nerve cells)

Where It's Found
Vegetables, beans, grains, and fortified cereals

Daily Dose
400 mcg

Can Be Used for (in Higher Doses)
Preventing developmental problems in babies (taken by mother before conception and during pregnancy)

What Happens If You Are Deficient?
Anemia, memory trouble, numbness and tingling, fatigue, and mouth sores

What Happens If You Take Too Much?
Excessive amounts of folic acid mask B12 deficiency so the neurological issues with B12 can progress without obvious findings in bloodwork

I Dine with Iodine

Iodine is a trace mineral to help with metabolism. It is a vitamin that is essential for our thyroid to function properly and make thyroid hormone.

Worldwide, iodine deficiency is the number one cause of goiters and hypothyroidism. In the 1920s, the United States actually started an iodized salt program in an effort to eliminate the risk of goiter and hypothyroidism in higher-risk areas. UNICEF has been spearheading a worldwide iodized-salt program since the 1990s. The intake of iodized salt has helped reduce these conditions.

The recommended daily allowance of iodine is 150 mcg. There are a number of natural sources of iodine in our diets. These sources include dairy products, saltwater fish, shellfish, soymilk, soy sauce, and seaweed. While many Americans are receiving the recommended level of iodine in their diets, some people, especially those on a low-salt diet, have lowered the amounts of iodine that they ingest. Some multivitamins contain the recommended amount of iodine, while many do not contain any at all. Pregnant and nursing women require even more iodine: 220 mcg and 290 mcg daily, respectively.

If many people need more iodine, should we all be taking it? And if so, how much? As many multivitamins don't include iodine, an extra supplement can be a good thing. However, many iodine supplements that are touted to help with thyroid support contain hundreds to thousands of times the recommended dosing (they are dosed in milligrams, not micrograms). These excessive amounts of iodine can actually cause hyperthyroidism! Too much iodine can cause your thyroid to "flare-up," leading to palpitations and anxiety. It could even lead to heart arrhythmias and osteoporosis among other serious medical conditions.

Iodine Highlights

What It Does
Helps cells with metabolism; used by the thyroid to create thyroid hormone

Where It's Found
Iodized salt, seafood, seaweed, soymilk, soy sauce, and dairy products

Daily Dose
150–290 mcg

Can Be Used for (in Higher Doses)
Thyroid support

What Happens If You Are Deficient?
Hypothyroidism/goiter (low metabolism, fatigue, weight gain, hair loss, and constipation)

What Happens If You Take Too Much?
Thyroid inflammation, hyperthyroidism (anxiety, palpitations, diarrhea, heart arrhythmias, and osteoporosis)

Invincible Iron

We grew up watching the *Popeye* cartoon. The somewhat goofy sailor guy would ingest massive quantities of spinach, and due to the iron he would gain mythical powers and strength. Frankly, the scenario holds some truth. We all need iron to function to our body's best ability. However, iron's role is more important to our overall energy than it is to actually building muscles. That technicality aside, replenishing iron in someone who is depleted can make them feel as exuberant as Popeye after a big dose of spinach.

Why is iron so important? Iron is used by your body to hold on to oxygen in your blood and transport it to your tissues. Iron is one of the key components in hemoglobin, the substance our red blood cells use to carry oxygen. At the cellular level, iron is used then to make energy and to fuel enzymes. Needless to say, any lack of iron has profound consequences on every aspect of the body.

Perhaps the most typical indication of a low level of iron is lack of energy. People often feel tired, sleepy, weak, "foggy," and short of breath. In severe cases of anemia (low red blood cell counts), people can have chest pain or pass out. Iron deficiency can also cause subtler symptoms, such as thinning hair (the body responds to what it perceives as a stressful situation by conserving its resources and not growing hair), or a condition called restless leg syndrome (where one gets tingling and a restless feeling in the legs that can profoundly interfere with sleep). Also associated with iron deficiency is an unusual tingling of the tongue, pain of the tongue, and something called pica, where people crave ice or unusual non-food items like ash, chalk, and clay. Clearly, iron is important to our bodies, and the body reacts to not having enough of it in a variety of ways.

Iron deficiency to a range of degrees is a very common issue today, particularly in women. Women's bodies are constantly shifting and changing. Iron loss is a normal part of this cycle. We require more iron during pregnancy and while nursing our children. Those who get menstrual periods, regularly lose blood and iron with menstruation. Heavier periods account for even more iron loss. All of these factors add up. Childbearing and monthly menses can deplete women's iron stores for years to follow.

Men too can be iron deficient due to less iron in their diets. In some instances, men or women can have unknown (or "occult") blood losses through their GI tracts, such as bleeding ulcers or bleeding colon polyps. These issues need to be addressed by a physician.

What is deceptive is that many people (and their doctors) do not realize they are iron deficient. Routine blood testing usually includes a CBC. This includes the hemoglobin and hematocrit levels, which reveal the amount of cells that are made from iron and are used by the blood to transport iron all over the body. Low hemoglobin or hematocrit are known as anemia, which is often the result of severe iron deficiency. Earlier stages of iron deficiency require special testing of specific iron and ferritin levels, which reflect how much iron your body has stored up.

While blood testing is useful, it is rarely essential. Our experience is that most premenopausal (and many postmenopausal) women can benefit from iron replacement to various degrees. In our experience, it is rare that someone's total body iron stores are up to snuff.

Then how do we replace the iron? Some of us replenish our iron from a well-rounded diet. However, the American diet has changed significantly over the last few decades. Our "healthier diet," geared toward prevention of heart disease, now contains significantly less red meat than it once did. Most of us are eating red meat on much rarer occasion than we used to. Fabulous as this may be for our cholesterol and heart health, it has actually contributed to widespread iron deficiency. Likewise, many processed foods are fortified with iron, but as we turn toward more whole and unprocessed foods we lose those sources.

While some vegetables, beans, and nuts do contain iron sources, they have lower amounts and are not as well absorbed. Therefore, vegetarians are at high risk for iron deficiency. Contributing to this confusion are antacids and anti-reflux medications, which can also decrease the absorption of the iron you do ingest. That means you may not actually be getting credit for the iron that you do take.

Finding the right iron-containing supplement can be a challenge. The downside of iron supplements is they often cause an upset stomach or constipation. The most common forms of iron supplements are ferrous sulfate and ferrous gluconate. It has been our experience that these forms are typically the worst GI offenders. At Vous Vitamin®, we worked hard to find the optimal form of iron to include in our supplements. We exclusively use iron in the form of carbonyl due to its superior absorption and better tolerability. Our customers give us great feedback on our multivitamins, many stating it is the first vitamin with iron that has not upset their stomachs.

One key element not to be overlooked with iron is optimizing its absorption. It turns out that iron needs to be taken with vitamin C in order for the GI tract to properly absorb it into the bloodstream and then incorporate it into cells. Therefore, when taking a separate iron supplement it should either be taken with foods high in C (a glass of orange juice will generally do) or in combination with a vitamin C supplement. Many multivitamins, including ours at Vous Vitamin®, take this into account and pair the two vitamins.

As with other nutrients, too much iron can be dangerous, and we advise caution in taking a supplement as it is intended to be taken. All vitamins containing iron are required to have a childproof cap, because iron in excess can actually be fatal. That is of course true only for very large doses. However, a small subset of the population has a condition called hemochromatosis. These people cannot handle even minimal doses of excess iron because it accumulates in their bodies. It then deposits in different organs and can cause liver damage or diabetes among other things. This is a genetic disorder that can be tested for. It is rare but illustrates to us how too much of any substance in the body can ultimately cause harm.

For these reasons, finding only the proper iron source in the correct amount is essential. It is also important to find the right means of absorbing that iron to feel more energetic and less fatigued. Iron replacement done right will build back levels over a few months' time and energy can return.

Iron Highlights

What It Does

Holds on to oxygen in your blood and transports it to your tissues

Where It's Found

Red meat, beans, lentils, and spinach

Daily Dose

15–28 mg daily (more to build up after losses)

Can Be Used for (in Higher Doses)

Energy, anemia, and fatigue

What Happens If You Are Deficient?

Lack of energy, hair loss, and shortness of breath

What Happens If You Take Too Much?

Upset stomach and constipation (at lower levels) and fatality (at overdose levels)

Magnificent Magnesium

Magnesium is one of our favorite vitamins. It is one of the few metals that many of us benefit from supplementing on a regular basis. We have seen many of our patients' health improve from taking magnesium for a variety of conditions.

Magnesium is an element that is in fact found in many different foods. However, many of us remain chronically low in magnesium. This is in part due to the fact that our food supply contains lower levels of certain nutrients than in the past due to soil demineralization and poor farming practices.

Magnesium is important to just about every aspect of bodily function. It serves to regulate the way cells work. It is essential for the working of muscles, building of bones, firing of nerves, cardiovascular function, and production of energy. Magnesium also plays a key role in potassium and calcium regulation.

Magnesium is found in many fruits and vegetables (bananas, greens, nuts, soy products, and whole grains). The U.S. RDA for magnesium intake is 320 to 420 mg daily. However, it is our experience that many people need more than this amount to maintain normal serum levels and to feel their best. People with gastrointestinal disease, alcoholism, or other malabsorption problems are more likely to have severe magnesium deficiency.

Deficiency in magnesium has been associated with migraines, osteoporosis, muscle aches, hypertension, and diabetes. Too much magnesium can cause serious neurological problems. It is rare, except in those with chronic kidney disease or those taking massive doses.

There is evidence to support supplemental magnesium's use for preventing and treating chronic migraines; preventing diabetes and improving glucose control; aiding in control of blood pressure; and helping with muscle aches or cramps, PMS, and sleep trouble. We have also found it to be very helpful in those with IBS. All around, we find magnesium to be a magnificent supplement. Of course, as with many supplements, it needs to be used in proper doses to ensure safety.

Magnesium Highlights

What It Does
Helps cells function properly; also involved in regulation of potassium and calcium

Where It's Found
Bananas, nuts, greens, soy, and whole grains

Daily Dose
320–420 mg is the U.S. RDA; many need more than they get via food

Can Be Used for (in Higher Doses)
Migraines, PMS, sleep, mood, blood pressure, muscle aches, and IBS

What Happens If You Are Deficient?
Weakness, fatigue, poor bone density, constipation, and headaches

What Happens If You Take Too Much?
Kidney and neurological problems

Oh My Omega-3s

There has been a great deal of talk about omega-3s and their potential health benefits. These essential fatty acids are nutrients that are useful for a lot of bodily functions. They play an important role in the prevention of blood clotting as well as in the formation of cell membranes, which help the brain function.

Omega-3s have been suggested to help reduce inflammation from a variety of conditions, including arthritis and IBD (such as Crohn's). They are recommended for some eye conditions such as macular degeneration. They have also been used for boosting mood and treating various neurological conditions, such as ADD.

Omega-3s can be found in both some vegetable sources and fish. Salmon, tuna, anchovies, or mackerel are great sources, as are canola oil, soybean oil, walnuts, and flaxseeds. Plant-based omega-3s are naturally converted by your body into the type of omega-3s found in fish (DHA and EPA). Fish oil supplements are a common way to ensure adequate intake of omega-3s.

Omega-3 supplements have good data to show that they are useful for reducing triglyceride levels (see the Cholesterol chapter) and may play a role in heart health and stroke prevention. They are also a standard recommendation during pregnancy. The role of fatty acids in neural development is felt to be important to fetal neurological growth.

When selecting a fish oil supplement, it is important to avoid high mercury levels, which is best done by sticking with a reputable brand. It is also important not to take excessive doses (2–3 grams per day maximum) as too much fish oil can cause excessive bleeding due to impaired blood clotting. In theory, high doses of fish oil can also cause impaired immune function.

We believe fish oil can be a useful supplement for some people. It can be useful for a variety of inflammatory conditions and/or vascular problems, and many feel it is helpful for memory, attention, and more. However, it should be used cautiously given that taking too much can have consequences.

Omega-3 Highlights

What It Does
Builds cell membranes and helps with nerve function

Where It's Found
Fish, vegetable oils, walnuts, and flaxseed

Daily Dose
1,000 mg

Can Be Used for (in Higher Doses)
Lowering triglycerides, ADD, and inflammation

What Happens If You Are Deficient?
Inflammatory illnesses and high triglycerides

What Happens If You Take Too Much?
Excess bleeding and immune dysfunction

Zealous About Zinc

Zinc is another elemental mineral that is an essential nutrient. It is found throughout the body and seems to play an important role in immunity and wound healing. Zinc is a key vitamin at certain times, particularly at the start of a respiratory infection.

Zinc is found in many high-protein foods, including meat, dairy, nuts, and legumes. Because of these many potential sources for zinc, most Americans are not deficient. However, those with certain malabsorption syndromes (like with IBD or after intestinal surgeries) may be deficient. The U.S. RDA is 9–13 mg daily.

Those deficient in zinc can suffer from immune deficiency, poor wound healing, and diarrhea. Conversely, zinc can be used to treat immune-related issues, in particular the common cold. It can be taken to promote wound healing and possibly prevent progression of macular degeneration (though data is conflicting on this). There is good data to suggest that taking zinc at the onset of cold symptoms can shorten the severity and duration of the infection. (See more in the Immunity chapter.)

It is our belief that zinc is useful at certain times for certain purposes; but it is rarely a daily necessity, given its abundance in the typical diet. At Vous Vitamin®, zinc is one of the key components of our Immune Blast™ supplement for this reason. We find it is useful when in need of extra immune support, such as when coming down with a cold or after exposure to an infection.

Excess intake of zinc can have negative effects such as GI upset, including nausea and vomiting. It can also cause urinary tract problems and neurological issues. Zinc in the proper doses (we believe no more than 100 mg daily) on select occasions can be a useful vitamin.

Zinc Highlights

What It Does
Helps T cells (or T lymphocytes) protect immunity and support wound healing

Where It's Found
Meat, oysters, dairy, nuts, whole grains, and legumes

Daily Dose
9–13 mg

Can Be Used For (in Higher Doses)
Colds, respiratory infections, wounds, and prevention of macular degeneration

What Happens If You Are Deficient?
Immune system problems and poor wound healing

What Happens If You Take Too Much?
Nausea, vomiting, low copper levels, and urinary problems

That's the A to Z on vitamins. We hope we have debunked the myths and shed light on how we all can use vitamins to support our well-being. Following are a list of references and resources you may find helpful as you continue to explore a healthier lifestyle.

REFERENCES AND RESOURCES

CHAPTER 1

"The Scientific 7-Minute Workout," Reynolds, G. *The New York Times*, May 9, 2013. Available online at: http://www.nytimes.com/compendium/reader/TVKRHBXQ74MGMEMYSM2IEVLKVP4/779/2710.

CHAPTER 2

"Vitamin and Mineral Supplements in the Primary Prevention of Cardiovascular Disease and Cancer: An Updated Systematic Evidence Review from the U.S. Preventative Services Task Force." Fortmann, S., et al. *Annals of Internal Medicine*, December 17, 2013; Vol. 159 (No. 12): 824–834.

"Long-Term Multivitamin Supplementation and Cognitive Function in Men: A Randomized Trial." Grodstein, F., et al. *Annals of Internal Medicine*, December 17, 2013; Vol. 159 (No. 12): 806–814.

"Vitamin, Mineral, and Multivitamin Supplements to Prevent Cardiovascular Disease and Cancer: Recommendations from the U.S. Preventative Services Task Force." *Annals of Internal Medicine*, April 15, 2014; Vol. 160 (No. 8): 1–24.

"The Effect of Vitamin E and Beta Carotene on the Incidence of Lung Cancer and Other Cancers in Male Smokers." The Alpha-Tocopherol, Beta Carotene Cancer Prevention Study Group. *New England Journal of Medicine*, April 14, 1994; Vol. 330 (No. 15): 1029–1035.

"Lead in Women's and Children's Vitamins." Mindak, W., et al. *Journal of Agricultural and Food Chemistry*, August 2008, Vol. 56 (No. 16): 6892–6896.

"Agriculture and Food: FDA Regulation of Dietary Supplements." July 2, 1993; HRD-93-28R. Available online at: http://www.gao.gov/products/HRD-93-28R.

"Herbal Dietary Supplements: Examples of Deceptive or Questionable Marketing Practices and Potentially Dangerous Advice." May 26, 2010; GAO-10-662T. Available online at: http://www.gao.gov/products/GAO-10-662T.

"Vitamin D: Fact Sheet for Health Professionals." National Institutes of Health, Office of Dietary Supplements. Available online at: http://ods.od.nih.gov/factsheets/VitaminD-HealthProfessional/.

"Iodine: Fact Sheet for Health Professionals." National Institutes of Health, Office of Dietary Supplements. Available online at: http://ods.od.nih.gov/factsheets/Iodine-HealthProfessional/.

"Alcohol Alert: Alcohol and Nutrition." National Institutes of Health, National Institute on Alcohol Abuse and Alcoholism, October 1993; No. 22. PH 346. Available online at: http://pubs.niaaa.nih.gov/publications/aa22.htm.

"Vitamin C for Preventing and Treating the Common Cold." Hemilä, H. and E. Chalker. *Cochrane Reviews*, January 31, 2013; 1: CD000980.

"New York Attorney General Targets Supplements at Major Retailers." O'Connor, A. *The New York Times*, February 3, 2015.

CHAPTER 3

"Vitamin D: Fact Sheet for Health Professionals." National Institutes of Health, Office of Dietary Supplements. Available online at: http://ods.od.nih.gov/factsheets/VitaminD-HealthProfessional/.

"Safety Issues Associated with Commercially Available Energy Drinks." Clauson, K.A., et al., *Journal of the American Pharmacists Association*, May–June 2008; Vol. 48 (No. 3): e55–63.

CHAPTER 4

"Iron: Dietary Supplement Fact Sheet." National Institutes of Health, Office of Dietary Supplements. Available online at: http://ods.od.nih.gov/factsheets/Iron-HealthProfessional/.

"Vitamin D Deficiency: A Worldwide Problem with Health Consequences." Holick, M.F. and T.C. Chen. *American Journal of Clinical Nutrition*, April 2008; Vol. 87 (No. 4): 10805–10865.

"Vitamin D: Fact Sheet for Health Professionals." National Institutes of Health, Office of Dietary Supplements. Available online at: http://ods.od.nih.gov/factsheets/VitaminD-HealthProfessional/.

"Vitamin B6: Dietary Supplement Fact Sheet." National Institutes of Health, Office of Dietary Supplements. Available online at: http://ods.od.nih.gov/factsheets/VitaminB6-HealthProfessional/.

"Vitamin B12: Dietary Supplement Fact Sheet." National Institutes of Health, Office of Dietary Supplements. Available online at: http://ods.od.nih.gov/factsheets/VitaminB12-HealthProfessional/.

"Iodine Supplementation for Pregnancy and Lactation—United States and Canada: Recommendations of the American Thyroid Association." Becker, D.V., et al. *Thyroid*, October 2006; Vol. 16 (No. 10): 949–951.

"Iodine: Fact Sheet for Health Professionals." National Institutes of Health, Office of Dietary Supplements. Available online at: http://ods.od.nih.gov/factsheets/Iodine-HealthProfessional/.

"Magnesium: Fact Sheet for Health Professionals." National Institutes of Health, Office of Dietary Supplements. Available online at: http://ods.od.nih.gov/factsheets/Magnesium-HealthProfessional/.

CHAPTER 5

Migraine Headache References and Support. Available online at: http://www.americanheadachesociety.org/.

Cleveland Clinic Migraine Center. Available online at: http://my.clevelandclinic.org/disorders/migraine_headache/hic_migraine_headaches.aspx.

"Role of Magnesium in the Pathogenesis and Treatment of Migraine." Sun-Edelstein, C. and A. Mauskop. *Expert Review Neurotherapeutics*, March 2009; Vol. 9 (No. 3): 369–379.

"Alternative Therapies in Headache. Is There a Role?" [Review]. Mauskop, A. *Medical Clinics of North America*, 2001; Vol. 85 (No. 4): 1077–1084.

Vitamin B2 (Riboflavin). University of Maryland Medical Center. Available online at: http://umm.edu/health/medical/altmed/supplement/vitamin-b2-riboflavin.

Vitamin B12: Dietary Supplement Fact Sheet." National Institutes of Health, Office of Dietary Supplements. Available online at: http://ods.od.nih.gov/factsheets/VitaminB12-HealthProfessional.

"Alcohol Alert: Alcohol and Nutrition." National Institutes of Health, National Institute on Alcohol Abuse and Alcoholism. October 1993; No. 22. PH 346. Available online at: http://pubs.niaaa.nih.gov/publications/aa22.htm.

CHAPTER 6

"Serum Ferritin and Vitamin D in Female Hair Loss: Do They Play a Role?" Rasheed, H., et al. *Skin Pharmacololgy and Physiology*, 2013; Vol. 26 (No. 2): 101–107.

"Iron-Deficiency Anemia." American Society of Hematology. Available online at: http://www.hematology.org/Patients/Anemia/Iron-Deficiency.aspx.

"Taking Iron Supplements." MedlinePlus. Available online at: http://www.nlm.nih.gov/medlineplus/ency/article/007478.htm.

"The Nonskeletal Effects of Vitamin D: An Endocrine Society Scientific Statement." Rosen, C., et al. *Endocrine Reviews*, June 2012; Vol. 33 (No. 3): 456–492.

"Evidence for Supplemental Treatments in Androgenetic Alopecia." Famenini, S. and C. Goh. *Journal of Drugs in Dermatology,* July 2014; Vol. 13 (No. 7): 809–812.

CHAPTER 7

"Vitamin D and the Omega-3 Fatty Acids Control Serotonin Synthesis and Action, Part 2: Relevance for ADHD, Bipolar, Schizophrenia, and Impulsive Behavior." Patrick, R.P. and B.N. Ames. *The Journal of the Federation of American Societies for Experimental Biology (The FASEB Journal)*. February 24, 2015, pii: fj. 14-268342.

"Efficacy of Supplementary Vitamins C and E on Anxiety, Depression and Stress in Type 2 Diabetic Patients: A Randomized, Single-Blind, Placebo-Controlled Trial." Mazloom, Z., et al. *Pakistan Journal of Biological Sciences*, November 15, 2013; Vol. 16 (No. 22): 1597–1600.

"Treatment of Depression: Time to Consider Folic Acid and Vitamin B12." Coppen, A. and C. Bolander-Gouaille. *Journal of Psychopharmacology*, January 2005; Vol. 19 (No. 1): 59–65.

"Formulations of Dietary Supplements and Herbal Extracts for Relaxation and Anxiolytic Action: Relarian." Weeks, B.S. *Medical Science Monitor*, November 2009; Vol. 15 (No. 11): RA256-262.

CHAPTER 8

"Irritable Bowel Syndrome." National Institute of Diabetes and Digestive and Kidney Diseases. (NIDDK). Available online at: http://www.niddk.nih.gov/health-information/health-topics/digestive-diseases/irritable-bowel-syndrome/Pages/overview.aspx.

"Efficacy and Safety of a Magnesium Sulfate–Rich Natural Mineral Water for Patients with Functional Constipation." Dupont, C., et al. *Clinical Gastroenterology Hepatology*, August 2014; Vol. 12 (No. 8): 1280–1287.

"Alteration of Gut Microbiota and Efficacy of Probiotics in Functional Constipation." Choi, C.H. and S. K. Chang. *Journal of Neurogastroenterology and Motility,* January 31, 2015; Vol. 21 (No. 1): 4–7.

"Efficacy of Prebiotics, Probiotics, and Synbiotics in Irritable Bowel Syndrome and Chronic Idiopathic Constipation: Systematic Review and Meta-Analysis." Ford, A.C., et al. *The American Journal of Gastroenterology*, October 2014; Vol. 109 (No. 10): 1547–1561.

CHAPTER 9

"Questions and Answers about the WHI Postmenopausal Hormone Therapy Trials." National Institutes of Health, Department of Health and Human Services, Women's Health Initiative. Available online at: http://www.nhlbi. nih.gov/whi/whi_faq.htm.

"Effects of Hormone Therapy on Cognition and Mood." Fischer, B., et al. *Fertility and Sterility*, April 2014; Vol. 101 (No. 4): 898–904.

"Hormone Therapy Use and Outcomes in the Women's Health Initiative Trials." Roehm, E. *The Journal of the American Medical Association (JAMA)*, January 22 and 29, 2014; Vol. 311 (No. 4): 417.

"Menopausal Hormone Therapy and Health Outcomes during the Intervention and Extended Poststopping Phases of the Women's Health Initiative Randomized Trials." Manson, J.E., et al. *The Journal of the American Medical Association (JAMA)*, October 2, 2013; Vol. 310 (No. 13): 1353–1368.

"Risks and Benefits of Estrogen Plus Progestin in Healthy Postmenopausal Women: Principal Results from the Women's Health Initiative Randomized Controlled Trial." Rossouw, J.E., et al. *The Journal of the American Medical Association (JAMA)*, July 17, 2002; Vol. 288 (No. 3): 321–333.

"Compounded Bioidentical Menopausal Hormone Therapy." American College of Obstetricians and Gynecologists Committee on Gynecologic Practice and American Society for Reproductive Medicine Practice Committee. *Fertility and Sterility*, August 2012; Vol. 98 (No. 2): 308–312.

"Committee Opinion No. 532: Compounded Bioidentical Menopausal Hormone Therapy." Committee on Gynecologic Practice and the American Society for Reproductive Medicine Practice Committee. *Obstetrics and Gynecology*, August 2012; Vol. 120: 411–415.

"Role of Androgens in Women's Sexual Dysfunction." Basson, R., et al. *Menopause*, September–October 2010; Vol. 17 (No. 5): 962–971.

"Non-Hormonal Management of Vasomotor Symptoms." Sassarini, J. and M. A. Lumsden. *Climacteric*, August 2013; Vol. 16, No. Supplement 1: 31–36.

"Hormonal and Nonhormonal Treatment of Vasomotor Symptoms." Krause, M.S. and S.T. Nakamimi. *Obstetrics and Gynecology Clinics of North America*, March 2015; Vol. 42 (No. 1): 163–179.

"Complementary and Alternative Medications for Women's Health Issues." Lloyd, K.B. and L.B. Hornsby, *Nutrition in Clinical Practice*. October–November 2009; Vol. 24 (No. 5): 589–608.

"Phytoestrogens for Menopausal Vasomotor Symptoms." Lethaby, A., et al. *Cochrane Database Systematic Reviews*, December 10, 2013; Vol. 12: CD001395.

"Dehydroepiandrosterone Sulfate and Postmenopausal Women." Goel, R.M. and A. R. Cappola. *Current Opinion in Endocrinology, Diabetes and Obesity*, June 2011; Vol. 18 (No. 3): 171–176.

"Ginseng, Sex Behavior, and Nitric Oxide." Murphy, L.L. and T.J. Tee. *Annals of New York Academy of Sciences*, May 2002; Vol. 962 (No. 1): 372–377.

CHAPTER 10

"Thyroid Disease Symptoms & Conditions: Information for Patients and Public." American Thyroid Association. Available online at: http://www.thyroid.org/patient-thyroid-information/thyroid-disease-symptoms/.

"Thyroid Disorders." Hormone Health Network. Available online at: http://www.hormone.org/diseases-and-conditions/thyroid.

"Thyroid Hormone Replacement Therapy." Wiersinga, W.M. *Hormone Research*, 2001; Vol. 56 (Supplement 1): 74–81.

"American Thyroid Association Statement on the Potential Risks of Excess Iodine Ingestion and Exposure." American Thyroid Association. June 5, 2013. Available online at: http://www.thyroid.org/ata-statement-on-the-potential-risks-of-excess-iodine-ingestion-and-exposure/.

"Iodine Deficiency." American Thyroid Association. June 4, 2012. Available online at: http://www.thyroid.org/iodine-deficiency/.

"Does Selenium Supplementation Affect Thyroid Function? Results from a Randomized, Controlled, Double-Blinded Trial in a Danish Population." Winther, K.H., et al. *European Journal of Endocrinology*, March 4, 2015; pii: EJE-15-0069.

"Selenium Supplementation for Patients with Graves' Hyperthyroidism (the GRASS Trial): Study Protocol for a Randomized Controlled Trial." Watt, T., et al. *Trials*, April 30, 2013; Vol. 14: 119.

"Myth vs. Fact: Adrenal Fatigue." Hormone Health Network, The Endocrine Society. Available online at: http://www.hormone.org/hormones-and-health/myth-vs-fact/adrenal-fatigue.

"Is There Such a Thing as Adrenal Fatigue?" Nippoldt, T. Mayo Clinic. Available online at: http://www.mayoclinic.org/diseases-conditions/addisons-disease/expert-answers/adrenal-fatigue/faq-20057906.

CHAPTER 11

"Questions and Answers: NIH Glucosamine/Chondroitin Arthritis Intervention Trial Primary Study." Available online at: http://nccih.nih.gov/research/results/gait/qa.htm.

"Drugs and Supplements: SAMe." Mayo Clinic, Patient Care and Health Info. Available online at: http://www.mayoclinic.org/drugs-supplements/same/safety/hrb-20059935.

"Vitamin C for Preventing and Treating the Common Cold." Hemilä, H. and E. Chalker. *Cochrane Reviews.* January 31, 2013; Vol. 1: CD000980.

"Vitamin C: Fact Sheet for Health Professionals." National Institutes of Health, Office of Dietary Supplements. http://ods.od.nih.gov/factsheets/VitaminC-HealthProfessional/.

"Inhibition of TLR8- and TLR4-induced Type 1 IFN Induction by Alcohol Is Different from Its Effects on Inflammatory Cytokine Production in Monocytes." Pang, M., et al. *BMC Immunology*, September 30, 2011; Vol. 12: 55.

CHAPTER 12

"Women Trying to Conceive Should Take Vitamins: Researchers." Smith, R. *The Telegraph*, December 2, 2011. Available online at: http://www.telegraph.co.uk/news/health/news/8928234/Women-trying-to-conceive-should-take-vitamins-researchers.html.

"Vitamin D Deficiency Linked to Reduced Pregnancy Rates." Paffoni, A. *Journal of Clinical Endocrinology and Metabolism*, August 18, 2014; DOI: 10.1210/jc.2014-1802. Available online at: http://www.healio.com/endocrinology/bone-mineral-metabolism/news/online/%7Bdbf47b5a-a432-42c3-b5d0-b1dc96bd3c32%7D/vitamin-d-deficiency-linked-to-reduced-pregnancy-rates.

"American Academy of Pediatrics Recommendations on Iodine Nutrition during Pregnancy and Lactation." Leung, A.M., et al. *Pediatrics*, October 1, 2014; Vol. 134 (No. 4): e1282.

"Iodine Supplementation: For Pregnant and Breastfeeding Women." National Health and Medical Research Council Public Statement. Available online at: http://www.nhmrc.gov.au/_files_nhmrc/publications/attachments/new45_statement.pdf/.

"Prenatal Omega-3 Fatty Acids: Review and Recommendations." Jordan, R.G. *Journal of Midwifery and Women's Health*, November–December 2010; Vol. 55 (No. 6): 520–528.

CHAPTER 13

"The Important Role of Sleep in Metabolism." Copinschi, G., et al. *Frontiers of Hormone Research*. 2014; Vol. 42: 59–72.

"Effects of Poor and Short Sleep on Glucose Metabolism and Obesity Risk." Spiegel, K., et al. *Nature Reviews Endocrinology*, May 2009; Vol. 5 (No. 5): 253–261.

"The Impact of Sleep Deprivation on Food Desire in the Human Brain." Greer, S.M., et al. *Nature Communications*, August 6, 2013; Vol. 4, Article Number: 2259.

"Iron: Dietary Supplement Fact Sheets." National Institutes of Health, Office of Dietary Supplements. Available online at: http://ods.od.nih.gov/factsheets/Iron-HealthProfessional/.

"Melatonin and Sleep." National Sleep Foundation, Sleep Topics. Available online at: http://sleepfoundation.org/sleep-topics/melatonin-and-sleep.

Magnesium: Fact Sheet for Health Professionals." National Institutes of Health, Office of Dietary Supplements. Available online at: http://ods.od.nih.gov/factsheets/Magnesium-HealthProfessional/.

"Vitamin B12: Dietary Supplement Fact Sheet." National Institutes of Health, Office of Dietary Supplements. Available online at: http://ods.od.nih.gov/factsheets/VitaminB12-HealthProfessional/.

"Vitamin D: Fact Sheet for Health Professionals." National Institutes of Health, Office of Dietary Supplements. Available online at: http://ods.od.nih.gov/factsheets/VitaminD-HealthProfessional/.

"Black Cohosh: Fact Sheet for Health Professionals." National Institutes of Health, Office of Dietary Supplements. Available online at: http://ods.od.nih.gov/factsheets/BlackCohosh-HealthProfessional/.

CHAPTER 14

"Bone Health Basics: Get the Facts." National Osteoporosis Foundation, Learn About Osteoporosis. Available online at: http://nof.org/learn/basics.

"Are You at Risk?" National Osteoporosis Foundation. Available online at: http://nof.org/articles/2.

"FRAX® Identifying People at High Risk for Fracture: WHO Fracture Risk Assessment Tool, A New Clinical Tool for Informed Treatment Decisions." International Osteoporosis Foundation. Available online at: http://osteoporosis.org.za/general/downloads/FRAX-report-09.pdf.

"Calcium Content of Foods." University of California, San Francisco Medical Center. Available online at: http://www.ucsfhealth.org/education/calcium_content_of_selected_foods/.

"The Women's Health Initiative: Hormone Therapy and Calcium/Vitamin D Supplementation Trials." Cauley, J.A. *Current Osteoporosis Reports*, September 2013; Vol. 11 (No. 3): 171–178.

"Osteoporosis Prevention and Management: Nonpharmacologic and Lifestyle Options." Christianson, M.S. and W. Shen. *Clinical Obstetrics and Gynecology*, December 2013; Vol. 56 (No. 4): 703–710.

CHAPTER 15

"The Effect of Phosphatidylserine Containing Omega-3 Fatty-Acids on Attention-Deficit Hyperactivity Disorder Symptoms in Children: A Double-Blind Placebo-Controlled Trial, Followed by an Open-Label Extension." Manor, I., et al. *European Psychiatry*, July 2012; Vol. 27 (No. 5): 335–342.

"The Effects of Magnesium Physiological Supplementation on Hyperactivity in Children with Attention Deficit Hyperactivity Disorder (ADHD). Positive Response to Magnesium Oral Loading Test." Starobrat-Hermelin, B. and T. Kozielec. *Magnesium Research*, June 1997; Vol. 10 (No. 2): 149–156.

"Melatonin and Sleep." National Sleep Foundation, Sleep Topics. Available online at: http://sleepfoundation.org/sleep-topics/melatonin-and-sleep.

"St. John's Wort and Depression." National Institute of Health, National Center for Complementary and Integrative Health. Available online at: http://nccih.nih.gov/health/stjohnswort/sjw-and-depression.htm.

"Zinc: Fact Sheets for Professionals." National Institutes of Health, Office of Dietary Supplements. Available online at: http://ods.od.nih.gov/factsheets/Zinc-HealthProfessional/.

"Iron and Alzheimer's Disease: The Good, the Bad and the Ugly." Collingwood, J., et al. Alzheimer's Society. *The Journal of Quality Research in Dementia*, Issue 3. Available online at: http://alzheimers.org.uk/site/scripts/documents_info.php?documentID=306&pageNumber=6.

"Vitamin D: Fact Sheet for Health Professionals." National Institutes of Health, Office of Dietary Supplements. Available online at: http://ods.od.nih.gov/factsheets/VitaminD-HealthProfessional/.

"Vitamin B12: Fact Sheet for Health Professionals." National Institutes of Health, Office of Dietary Supplements. Available online at: http://ods.od.nih.gov/factsheets/VitaminB12-HealthProfessional/.

"The Role of Nutraceuticals in Dementia Care." Ford, J.M., et al. *Journal of Gerontological Nursing*, April 2014; Vol. 40 (No. 4): 11–17.

CHAPTER 16

"Hypertension among Adults in the United States, 2009–2010." Sug Yoon, S., et al. National Center for Health Statistics Data Brief, October 2012, No. 107. Available online at: http://www.cdc.gov/nchs/data/databriefs/db107.htm.

"Hypertension Guidelines." American Society of Hypertension. Available online at: http://www.ash-us.org/About-Hypertension/Hypertension-Guidelines.aspx.

"Effects of Exercise, Diet and Weight Loss on High Blood Pressure." Bacon, S.L., et al. *Sports Medicine*, 2004; Vol. 34 (No. 5): 307–316.

"Exercising Your Way to Better Blood Pressure." American College of Sports Medicine. Available online at: http://www.acsm.org/docs/brochures/exercising-your-way-to-lower-blood-pressure.pdf.

"Ask the Expert: Coffee and Health." van Dam, R. Harvard School of Public Health. Available online at: http://www.hsph.harvard.edu/nutritionsource/coffee/.

"How Smoking Affects Blood Pressure." Omvik, P. *Blood Press.* March 1996; Vol. 5 (No. 2): 71–77.

"Reducing Salt Intake for Prevention of Cardiovascular Disease—Times Are Changing." Stolarz-Skrzypek, K. and J. A. Staessen. *Advances in Chronic Kidney Disease*, March 2015; Vol. 22 (No. 2): 108–115.

"DASH Diet: Healthy Eating to Lower Your Blood Pressure." Mayo Clinic, Healthy Living. Available online at: http://www.mayoclinic.org/healthy-living/nutrition-and-healthy-eating/in-depth/dash-diet/art-20048456.

"Potassium Lowers Blood Pressure." Harvard Medical School. *Harvard Health Publications*. Available online at: http://www.health.harvard.edu/family_health_guide/potassium-lowers-blood-pressure.

Magnesium: Fact Sheet for Health Professionals." National Institutes of Health, Office of Dietary Supplements. Available online at: http://ods.od.nih.gov/factsheets/Magnesium-HealthProfessional/.

"Vitamin C: Fact Sheet for Health Professionals." National Institutes of Health, Office of Dietary Supplements. Available online at: http://ods.od.nih.gov/factsheets/VitaminC-HealthProfessional/.

"Big Doses of Vitamin C May Lower Blood Pressure: But Hold the Supplements, for Now, Researchers Say." John Hopkins Medicine, April 18, 2012. Available online at: http://www.hopkinsmedicine.org/news/media/releases/big_doses_of_vitamin_c_may_lower_blood_pressure.

"Effect on Blood Pressure of Potassium, Calcium, and Magnesium in Women with Low Habitual Intake." Sacks, F.M., et al. *Hypertension*, 1998; Vol. 31: 131–138.

CHAPTER 17

"What Your Cholesterol Levels Mean." American Heart Association. Available online at: http://www.heart.org/HEARTORG/Conditions/Cholesterol/AboutCholesterol/What-Your-Cholesterol-Levels-Mean_UCM_305562_Article.jsp.

"Metabolism of HDL and Its Regulation." Kardassis D, et al. *Current Medical Chemistry*, 2014; Vol. 21 (No. 25): 2864–2880.

"HDL Cholesterol: How to Boost Your 'Good' Cholesterol." Mayo Clinic, Diseases and Conditions, High Cholesterol. Available online at: http://www.mayoclinic.org/diseases-conditions/high-blood-cholesterol/in-depth/hdl-cholesterol/art-20046388?pg=1.

"Cholesterol-Lowering Effects of Dietary Fiber: A Meta-Analysis." Brown, L., et al. *American Journal of Clinical Nutrition*, January 1999; Vol. 69 (No. 1): 30–42.

"Incidence of Hospitalized Rhabdomyolysis in Patients Treated with Lipid-Lowering Drugs." Graham, D.J., et al. *The Journal of the American Medical Association (JAMA)*, December 1, 2004; Vol. 292 (No. 21): 2585–2590.

"Strategies to Preserve the Use of Statins in Patients with Previous Muscular Adverse Effects." Reinhart, K.M., et al. *American Journal of Health-System Pharmacy*, February 15, 2012: Vol. 69 (No. 4): 291–300.

"Red Yeast." National Institutes of Health, U.S. National Library of Medicine, Medline Plus. Available online at: http://www.nlm.nih.gov/medlineplus/druginfo/natural/925.html.

"Effect on Cardiovascular Risk of High Density Lipoprotein Targeted Drug Treatments Niacin, Fibrates, and CETP Inhibitors: Meta-Analysis of Randomised Controlled Trials Including 117,411 Patients." Keene, D., et al. *British Medical Journal*, July 18, 2014; Vol. 349: g4379.

"Bedside to Bench: The Risk of Bleeding with Parenteral Omega-3 Lipid Emulsion Therapy." Dicken, B.J., et al. *Journal of Pediatrics*, March 2014; Vol. 164 (No. 3): 652–654.

CHAPTER 18

"Type 2." American Diabetes Association, Diabetes Basics. Available online at: http://www.diabetes.org/diabetes-basics/type-2/?loc=db-slabnav.

"Low Vitamin D and Type 2 Diabetes: How Do Vitamin D Levels Correlate with HbA1c?" Diabetes in Control. Available online at: http://www.diabetesincontrol.com/articles/diabetes-news/15490-low-vitamin-d-and-type-2-diabetes.

"Efficacy of Alpha-Lipoic Acid in Diabetic Neuropathy." Papanas, N., et al. *Expert Opinion on Pharmacotherapy*, December 2014; Vol. 15 (No. 18): 2721–2731.

"Chromium Picolinate and Biotin Combination Improves Glucose Metabolism in Treated, Uncontrolled Overweight to Obese Patients with Type 2 Diabetes." Albarracin, C.A., et al. *Diabetes/Metabolism Research and Reviews*, January–February 2008; Vol. 24 (No. 1): 41–51.

"Cinnamon Use in Type 2 Diabetes: An Updated Systematic Review and Meta-Analysis." Allen, R.W., et al. *The Annals of Family Medicine*, September–October 2013; Vol. 11 (No. 5): 452–459.

"Role of Dietary Magnesium in Cardiovascular Disease Prevention, Insulin Sensitivity and Diabetes." Bo, S. and E. Pisu. *Current Opinions in Lipidology*, February 2008; Vol. 19 (No. 1): 50–56.

"The Prevalence of Low Vitamin B12 Status in People with Type 2 Diabetes Receiving Metformin Therapy in New Zealand: A Clinical Audit." Haeusler, S., et al. *New Zealand Medical Journal*, October 17, 2014; Vol. 127 (No. 1404): 8–16.

"Overall Numbers, Diabetes and Prediabetes." American Diabetes Association, Statistics About Diabetes. Released June 10, 2014. Available online at:http://www.diabetes.org/diabetes-basics/statistics/?loc=db-slabnav.

CHAPTER 19

"New Lung Cancer Screening Guidelines for Heavy Smokers." American Cancer Society, January 11, 2013. Available online at: http://www.cancer.org/cancer/news/new-lung-cancer-screening-guidelines-for-heavy-smokers.

"American Cancer Society Guidelines for the Early Detection of Cancer: Breast Cancer." American Cancer Society. Available online at: http://

www.cancer.org/healthy/findcancerearly/cancerscreeningguidelines/
american-cancer-society-guidelines-for-the-early-detection-of-cancer.

"Cervical Cancer Statistics." Center for Disease Control and Prevention. Available online at: http://www.cdc.gov/cancer/cervical/statistics/.

"Osteoporosis Screening." U.S. Preventive Services Task Force. Released January 2011. Available online at: http://www.uspreventiveservicestaskforce. org/Page/Topic/recommendation-summary/osteoporosis-screening.

American Cancer Society Guidelines for the Early Detection of Cancer: Colorectal Cancer and Polyps." Available online at: http:// www.cancer.org/healthy/findcancerearly/cancerscreeningguidelines/ american-cancer-society-guidelines-for-the-early-detection-of-cancer.

CHAPTER 20

"Weight Loss: Strategies for Success." Mayo Clinic, Healthy Lifestyle. Available online at: http://www.mayoclinic.org/healthy-living/weight-loss/in-depth/ weight-loss/art-20047752.

"7 Simple Changes That Will Help You Lose Weight." Weight Watchers. Available online at: http://www.weightwatchers.com/util/art/index_art. aspx?tabnum=1&art_id=771&sc=3046.

"Dietary Self-Monitoring, but Not Dietary Quality, Improves with Use of Smartphone App Technology in an 8-Week Weight Loss Trial." Wharton, C.M., et al. *Journal of Nutrition Education and Behavior*, September–October 2014; Vol. 46 (No. 5): 440–444.

South Beach Diet. Available online at: http://www.southbeachdiet.com/diet/.

"Over-the-Counter Weight-Loss Pills." Mayo Clinic, Healthy Lifestyle, Weight Loss. Available online at: http://www.mayoclinic.org/healthy-living/ weight-loss/in-depth/weight-loss/art-20046409.

"Does Glycine Max Leaves or Garcinia Cambogia Promote Weight-Loss or Lower Plasma Cholesterol in Overweight Individuals: A Randomized Control Trial." Kim, J.E., et al. *Nutrition Journal*, September 21, 2011; Vol. 10: 94.

"Questions and Answer on the HCG Products for Weight Loss." U.S. Food and Drug Administration, Food and Drug Administration. Available online at: http://www.fda.gov/Drugs/ResourcesForYou/Consumers/BuyingUsingMedicineSafely/MedicationHealthFraud/ucm281834.htm.

"Toxicity of Weight Loss Agents." Yen, M. and M. B. Ewald. *Journal of Medical Toxicology*, June 2012; Vol. 8 (No. 2): 145–152.

"Multi-ingredient, Caffeine-containing Dietary Supplements: History, Safety, and Efficacy." Gurley, B.J., et al. *Clinical Therapeutics*, February 1, 2015; Vol. 37 (No. 2): 275–301.

"An Analysis of Energy-Drink Toxicity in the National Poison Data System." Seifert, S.M., et al. *Clinical Toxicology*, August 2013; Vol. 51 (No. 7): 566–574.

CHAPTER 21

"How Much Physical Activity Do You Need?" Center for Disease Control and Prevention, Physical Activity. Available online at: http://www.cdc.gov/physicalactivity/everyone/guidelines/index.html.

"The Scientific 7-Minute Workout" Reynolds, G. *The New York Times*, May 9, 2013. Available online at: http://www.nytimes.com/compendium/reader/TVKRHBXQ74MGMEMYSM2IEVLKVP4/779/2710.

"Exercise-Induced AMPK Activation Does Not Interfere with Muscle Hypertrophy in Response to Resistance Training in Men." Lundberg, T.R., et al. *Journal of Applied Physiology*, March 15, 2014; Vol. 116 (No. 6): 611–620.

CHAPTER 22

"The New Food Pyramid." *The Washington Post*. Available online at: http://www.washingtonpost.com/wp-srv/nation/daily/graphics/diet_042005.html.

"Food Guide Pyramid." United States Department of Agriculture, Center for Nutrition Policy and Promotion. Available online at: http://www.cnpp.usda.gov/FGP.

"MyPlate Resources." United States Department of Agriculture, Center for Nutrition Policy and Promotion, Nutrition Information for You, Smart Nutrition 101. Available online at: http://www.nutrition.gov/smart-nutrition-101/myplate-food-pyramid-resources.

"Protein." Centers for Disease Control and Prevention, Nutrition for Everyone. Available online at: http://www.cdc.gov/nutrition/everyone/basics/protein. html.

"Carbohydrates." Centers for Disease Control and Prevention, Nutrition for Everyone. Available online at: http://www.cdc.gov/nutrition/everyone/basics/ carbs.html.

Celiac Disease and Gluten-free Diet Information. Available online at: http:// www.celiac.com.

"Is Organic Better for Your Health? A look at Milk, Meat, Eggs, Produce and Fish." Haspel, T. *The Washington Post*, Health and Science, April 7, 2014. Available online at: http://www.washingtonpost.com/national/health-science/ is-organic-better-for-your-health-a-look-at-milk-meat-eggs-produce-and- fish/2014/04/07/036c654e-a313-11e3-8466-d34c451760b9_story.html.

"Diet and Lifestyle Recommendations Revision 2006: A Scientific Statement from the American Heart Association Nutrition Committee." *Circulation*, July 4, 2006; Vol. 114 (No. 1): 82–96.

"Put Down That Doughnut: FDA Takes on Trans Fats." Hayes, A. CNN. November 13, 2013. Available online at: http://www.cnn.com/2013/11/07/ health/fda-trans-fats/.

"Association of Dietary, Circulating, and Supplement Fatty Acids with Coronary Risk: A Systematic Review and Meta-Analysis." Chowdhury, R., et al. *Annals of Internal Medicine*, March 18, 2014; Vol. 160 (No. 6): 398–406.

"Comparison of Prevalence of Inadequate Nutrient Intake Based on Body Weight Status of Adults in the United States: An Analysis of NHANES 2001– 2008." Agarwal, S., et al. *Journal of the American College of Nutrition*, January 2015; DOI: 10.1080/07315724.2014.

"Multivitamin-Mineral Use Is Associated with Reduced Risk of Cardiovascular Disease Mortality Among Women in the United States." Bailey, R.L., et al. *Journal of Nutrition*, March 2015; jn.114.204743.

VITAMIN GLOSSARY

"Vitamin A: Dietary Supplement Fact Sheets." National Institutes of Health, Office of Dietary Supplements. Available online at: http://ods.od.nih.gov/factsheets/VitaminA-HealthProfessional/.

"[Vitamin B1] Thiamin: Dietary Supplement Fact Sheet." National Institutes of Health, Office of Dietary Supplements. Available online at: http://ods.od.nih.gov/factsheets/Thiamin-HealthProfessional/.

"Vitamin B6 [Pyridoxine]: Dietary Supplement Fact Sheet." National Institutes of Health, Office of Dietary Supplements. Available online at: http://ods.od.nih.gov/factsheets/VitaminB6-HealthProfessional/.

"Vitamin B12: Dietary Supplement Fact Sheet." National Institutes of Health, Office of Dietary Supplements. Available online at: http://ods.od.nih.gov/factsheets/VitaminB12-HealthProfessional/.

"Vitamin C: Dietary Supplement Fact Sheet." National Institutes of Health, Office of Dietary Supplements. Available online at: http://ods.od.nih.gov/factsheets/VitaminC-HealthProfessional/.

"Calcium: Dietary Supplement Fact Sheet." National Institutes of Health, Office of Dietary Supplements. Available online at: http://ods.od.nih.gov/factsheets/Calcium-HealthProfessional/.

"Vitamin D: Dietary Supplement Fact Sheet." National Institutes of Health, Office of Dietary Supplements. Available online at: http://ods.od.nih.gov/factsheets/VitaminD-HealthProfessional/

"Vitamin E: Dietary Supplement Fact Sheet." National Institutes of Health, Office of Dietary Supplements. Available online at: http://ods.od.nih.gov/factsheets/VitaminE-HealthProfessional/.

"Iodine: Dietary Supplement Fact Sheet." National Institutes of Health, Office of Dietary Supplements. Available online at: http://ods.od.nih.gov/factsheets/Iodine-HealthProfessional/.

"Iron: Dietary Supplement Fact Sheet." National Institutes of Health, Office of Dietary Supplements. Available online at: http://ods.od.nih.gov/factsheets/Iron-HealthProfessional/.

"Magnesium: Dietary Supplement Fact Sheet." National Institutes of Health, Office of Dietary Supplements. Available online at: http://ods.od.nih.gov/factsheets/Magnesium-HealthProfessional/.

"Ask the Expert: Omega-3 Fatty Acids." Sacks, F. Harvard School of Public Health. Available online at: http://www.hsph.harvard.edu/nutritionsource/omega-3/.

"Zinc: Dietary Supplement Fact Sheet." National Institutes of Health, Office of Dietary Supplements. Available online at: http://ods.od.nih.gov/factsheets/Zinc-HealthProfessional/.

ACKNOWLEDGMENTS

WHEN TWO WOMEN PHYSICIANS—with busy practices and six kids under the age of eleven between them—say they are going to launch a business and then write a book in their "spare time," their husbands' natural response is not typically, "Great idea, honey." That was in fact the reaction from both of our husbands. And they meant it. And they continue to support us (to the best of their abilities) in all of our endeavors. For two six-foot-tall men, they make great cheerleaders. They first listened to our woes about the practice of medicine and its many imperfections, as well as our concerns about the way vitamins have been addressed (or not addressed) in our medical model. They then wholeheartedly embraced our desire to "do vitamins right." They have hauled boxes, driven carpools, attended events, and given us tremendous input (from their own years of medical practice) for the book. Our efforts may not meet their standards for classic Russian literature, but they can both agree that this book does not suck. In fact, we all hope it will be a useful guide.

And then there are our kids. In their own ways, they have, if nothing else, given us motivation, drive, and inspiration to make this project a reality. They have complained about their moms attending "another meeting" many times, but only to be elated when they see our products sitting on someone's kitchen counter. It is our sincere hope that they will look at what we have created and written, and be inspired to envision and forge their own new realities someday.

We would be remiss if we did not give a huge thank you to Steve and Robin Prebish for their roles in making both Vous Vitamin® and *The Vitamin Solution* come into being. Their tireless efforts behind the scenes have enabled us to both create a business and have the time and resources to write this book. They have been supportive, insightful, and the voices of reality at every step of the way. Likewise, we credit Wendi Ezgur with helping us "get real" when our idea was only an idea. Beth Richman has helped us get the word out about Vous Vitamin® and *The Vitamin Solution* in ways we did not know were possible, and for that we are grateful.

Next we must give great credit to Gina Bianchini and Kamy Wicoff for their inspiration. Who knew that two doctors could ever have the know-how to start a business and write a book? Apparently they did. Starting with our first summit in Gina's backyard, they ignited in us the courage to create a company and a book so we could share the knowledge we have obtained with anyone willing to read it. Gina is the pied piper of female entrepreneurship. Kamy taught us more than we wanted to know about the publishing industry and connected us with wonderful people like Annie Tucker and Brooke Warner at She Writes Press, who helped us distill vast amounts of knowledge obtained from years of practicing medicine and selling vitamins into book form. Annie patiently listened to the two of us debate about medical topics and helped us infuse life into reams of dry medical information. She also taught us that lay people do not know the meaning of terms such as "body habitus."

Last, but certainly not least, we must thank all of our patients and customers over the years who have given us stories to tell and endless insights into health and vitamins we could not have had otherwise.

ABOUT THE AUTHORS

Arielle Miller Levitan

Arielle Miller Levitan, MD, is a board-certified internal medicine physician and the cofounder of Vous Vitamin, LLC. She attended Stanford University and Northwestern University's Feinberg School of Medicine, and has served as chief medical resident for the Northwestern University McGaw Medical Center's Evanston Hospital Program and as a clinical instructor for its medical school. She has a special interest in women's health and preventive medicine and currently practices general internal medicine on the North Shore of Chicago, where she teaches medical students on-site. She enjoys cooking, cardio tennis, being a soccer mom (sometimes), and spending time with her three kids and husband (also a doctor of internal medicine).

Romy Block

Romy Block, MD, is a board-certified specialist in endocrine and metabolism medicine, and the cofounder of Vous Vitamin, LLC. She attended Tufts University and Tel Aviv University's Sackler School of Medicine. She completed residency training in internal medicine at North Shore University Hospital—North Shore-LIJ and did a fellowship at New York University. She practices on the North Shore of Chicago, where she specializes in thyroid disorders and pituitary diseases. She enjoys travel, food and wine, and spending time with her husband (a pulmonary and sleep specialist) and their three boys.